T0202860

Exercise
Testing in
Cardiology

Springer

Paris
Berlin
Heidelberg
New York
Hong Kong
London
Milan
Tokyo

Exercise Testing in Cardiology

Editorial coordination
Jean-Marc Foult

Bernard Attal
Alain Ducardonnet
Olivier Hoffman
Laurent Uzan
Jean-Claude Verdier
Pierre Weinmann

Foreword by Philippe Gabriel Steg

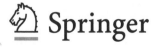 Springer

Bernard Attal
American Hospital of Paris
63, boulevard Victor-Hugo
92200 Neuilly-sur-Seine

Alain Ducardonnet
American Hospital of Paris
63, boulevard Victor-Hugo
92200 Neuilly-sur-Seine
Cœur Effort Santé Institut
36 bis, boulevard Saint-Marcel
75005 Paris

Jean-Marc Foult
American Hospital of Paris
63, boulevard Victor-Hugo
92200 Neuilly-sur-Seine

Olivier Hoffman
American Hospital of Paris
63, boulevard Victor-Hugo
92200 Neuilly-sur-Seine

Laurent Uzan
American Hospital of Paris
63, boulevard Victor-Hugo
92200 Neuilly-sur-Seine
Cœur Effort Santé Institut
36 bis, boulevard Saint-Marcel
75005 Paris

Jean-Claude Verdier
Cœur Effort Santé Institut
36 bis, boulevard Saint-Marcel
75005 Paris

Pierre Weinmann
Avicenne Hospital
25, rue de Stalingrad
93009 Bobigny Cedex

ISBN : 978-2-287-99498-2 Springer Paris Berlin Heidelberg New York
© Springer-Verlag France, Paris 2009

Springer-Verlag France is member of Springer Science + Business Media

*This publication has been made possible
through an educational grant from SERVIER*

Layout: Bloc images
Cover design: Jean-François Montmarché

Table of contents

Foreword

EXERCISE TESTING IN CARDIOLOGY IS MORE TOPICAL THAN EVER

Despite advances in noninvasive imaging that facilitate identification of coronary stenoses in asymptomatic patients or in patients with atypical symptoms, exercise testing is more crucial than ever in diagnostic and prognostic evaluation.

We now know that diagnostic strategies based solely on morphological identification of coronary stenoses are ineffective, costly, and cause iatrogenic complications.

COURAGE and similar studies of the role of revascularization in patients with stable coronary disease have shown that infarction and sudden death cannot be avoided by prophylactic dilation of tight coronary stenoses. Instead, what matters prognostically in a given patient is not so much the presence or even degree of coronary stenosis, but rather its physiological implications in terms of myocardial ischemia.

And for this, all the world's scanners are no substitute for a good exercise test, which all too often is requested after a scan has identified a stenosis in an asymptomatic patient. Exercise testing should be the first diagnostic technique used in patients suspected to have effort angina, and the demonstration of myocardial ischemia should precede the use of imaging techniques in identifying the causes in the coronary network.

Exercise testing also provides information that goes well beyond a simple positive test/negative test classification. The degree of effort reached, changes in blood pressure and heart rate, the size and type of electrocardiographic changes observed, how early these occur, their relation to symptoms, the presence and development of arrhythmia are all simple to identify and are decisive for the clinician's diagnostic and prognostic evaluation.

In the 21st century exercise testing is often no longer just a simple test, but rather has been considerably enhanced by coupling with isotopic techniques and blood gas analysis, which improve performance and yield more complete data.

The seasoned experts who describe all these techniques clearly and precisely in this valuable book are to be warmly thanked for the great service they have rendered clinicians everywhere.

Philippe Gabriel Steg

Department of Cardiology,
Bichat-Claude Bernard Hospital
Université Paris 7 – Denis Diderot.

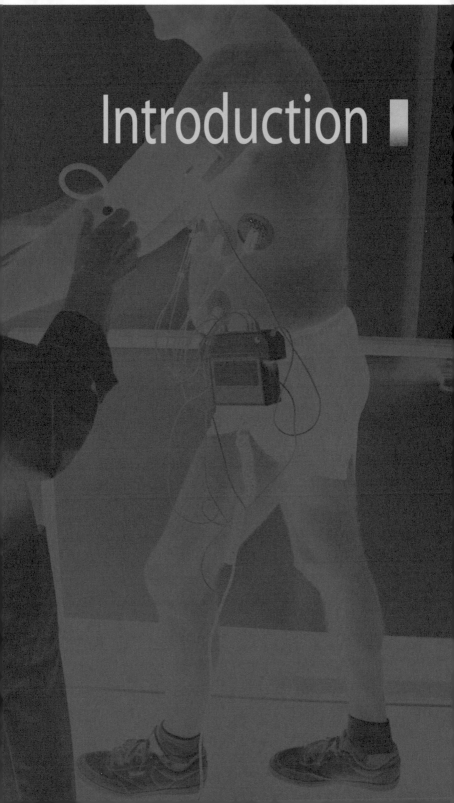

Introduction

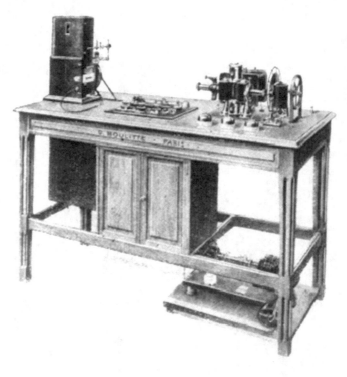

Fig. 1 - The first "cardiographic recording".

Introduction

EXERCISE TESTING:
A HEALTHY CENTENARIAN

T
he history of exercise testing covers a fascinating century during which it kept pace with technical innovations and progress, yet continually had its clinical relevance challenged. In medicine, as elsewhere, what can be done and what should be done are two separate notions: the capacity to do something is not proof of its clinical usefulness. Here, we will briefly recount the story of exercise testing, its advances and challenges.

When William Heberden wrote the first description of angina in 1768, he was aware that this symptom corresponded to the presence of atheromatous lesions of the coronary arteries. Research by illustrious pathologists at the time had proven that chest pain, which was intuitively attributed to the heart, did in fact correspond to coronary artery disease.

When speaking of exercise testing, we need to retrace a kind of "electrical history" of the heart. The story began with Luigi Galvani, who demonstrated that living tissues produce electrical activity. At the end of the nineteenth century, the French physiologist Étienne Jules Marey recorded the heart's electrical activity on the surface of the skin, and immediately afterwards, Willem Einthoven (of the future Einthoven's triangle) produced the first "cardiographic recording". Electrodes were placed on a patient's chest to measure the current, which set in motion a thin silver wire stretched between the poles of a large magnet. These deflections were recorded on photographic paper that unrolled in front of a light source. The electrocardiogram was born, making it possible to record the electrical activity of normal and diseased hearts. Today, it is difficult to imagine the impact of this discovery. Over the decades, thousands of publications were written, describing various leads, the different stages of the electrocardiographic cycle and their alterations in various diseases. These topics as well as cardiac rhythm disturbances were in the foreground until the 1970s.

In this flurry of activity came electrocardiographic signs of acute myocardial infarction. The discovery of ST-segment modifications (Pardee's wave), T wave, and then Q waves turned the world of cardiology upside down by making it possible to diagnose accurately one of the main scourges of the twentieth century.

Patients with suspected acute myocardial infarction were hospitalized and, consequently, the first reversible repolarization changes occurring during angina were recorded.

Yet angina is a symptom that more readily occurs during exercise. Could one take the risk of artificially triggering angina with supervised exercise? And was it technically possible to record an electrocardiogram under these conditions?

ANGINA, ELECTRICAL ACTIVITY OF THE HEART, AND EXERCISE:
THE SCENE IS SET

In 1908, Einthoven published the first electrocardiogram (ECG) recorded just after exercise, showing an ST depression. This was only a factual description without an interpretation, but the date is nevertheless traditionally considered to be the starting point of exercise testing.

For twenty years, this electrical modification - occurring during spontaneous angina or following exercise, with or without anginal pain - was mentioned in any number of published studies.

The sequence: exercise, appearance of ST depression, angina, interruption of the exercise, disappearance of pain, normalization of the ECG - hinted at what would later be known as the ischemic cascade.

Yet things were not that simple, and disagreements arose. Was it legitimate to voluntarily trigger an angina attack? Did this approach have real practical consequences for the patient or was it just an academic curiosity, not devoid of risk? Moreover, difficulties linked to ECG recording and the absence of standardized protocols fueled the debate.

1930 TO 1950
SEARCHING FOR AN IDENTITY

Arthur Master published the first standardized cardiac stress test in 1929. His aim was to assess the physical capacity of a subject who repeatedly climbed steps 22.9 cm high, and he had little concern for ECG and repolarization.

At the same time, cardiologists continued to document the relationship between exercise and repolarization changes. Goldhammer and Scherf were the first to quantify this link: they recorded a positive electrical charge in about 75% of patients with angina during exercise, which is similar to current percentages.

A short while afterwards, the CM5 lead was described as the most sensitive. Missal applied the Master test to diagnose angina. It was found that the ECG should be recorded as soon as possible after exercise ends, and that nitrates increase the pain threshold. In 1940, Riseman made a continuous ECG recording during the Master test. Working with Jaffe, Master confirmed the value of combining exercise and ECG. All the elements of exercise testing were now in place for the diagnosis of ischemia, and progressive refinements were made over the next fifteen years.

> From a technical point of view, it is difficult not to be struck by the lack of uniformity in how much exercise is required and its quality. In some cases, the test goes on until there is a painful crisis; in others, the test is less daring and is limited to moderate exercise. We believe a clinician who has sufficient documentation does not have the right to expose his patient to potentially dangerous accidents in the name of an interest that is often more documentary than practical, and we admit to remaining below the exercise levels needed to satisfy reckless curiosity. Therefore, among the exercises generally chosen (which would also benefit from standardization), we prefer climbing steps in a set time over other more tiring or vigorous activities such as pedaling and weightlifting.
>
> Translated excerpt from *Les maladies des coronaires*,
> Laubry and Soulié, Masson et Cie, 1943.

EXERCISE PROTOCOL, ASSESSMENT OF CHEST PAIN AND ST DEPRESSION:

THE ROAD TO STANDARDIZATION

Inspired by the Master test, Johnson developed the Harvard Step Test to assess aerobic fitness in relation to heart rates in athletes. This was the first time heart rate recovery was considered an index of good health. In 1951, these studies were extended to cardiac patients, leading to a broader impact on society. This was the beginning of cardiac rehabilitation, which aimed to promote a return to an active working and social life after a cardiovascular accident.

In ischemia, pain and ST depression only occur simultaneously in 50% of cases, while electrical recordings are clearly more sensitive. In the early 1950s, two publications summarized criteria that are now familiar.

▶ In 1950, Wood, in London, stipulated that:
- Exercise levels must be personalized;
- In coronary patients, a heart rate above 90 beats per min (sic) increases the number of positive tests;
- Climbing 84 steps (nearly a maximum test) increases reliability to about 90%, compared with 39% for the Master test.

▶ In 1952, Yu and Stewart published the following ECG criteria as positive (continuous ECG recording during the Master test):
- ST- segment depression greater than 1 mm;
- Negative T wave and/or return to positive;
- Increase in T wave amplitude of more than 50% compared with amplitude at rest (more controversial).

▶ In 1956, in Seattle, Robert A. Bruce set the exercise test standard: the test was performed on a treadmill with varying levels of difficulty based on New York Heart Disease classifications.

THE 1960s

THE 1960s WERE CHARACTERIZED BY A SERIES OF TECHNOLOGICAL CHANGES, DOMINATED BY PROGRESS MADE IN COMPUTER SCIENCE AND THE ADVENT OF CORONARY ANGIOGRAPHY.

Blackburn refined the criteria for ST-T changes in ischemia, and the CM5 and V5 leads proved of value. This simplification led to more widespread use of the technique. ST-segment depression in screening was shown to be of greater predictive value than clinical data. Bruce then standardized these criteria and introduced computers into exercise testing, using digital signals for ST-segment analysis.

The considerable development of coronary angiography gave exercise testing both a benchmark and justification of its clinical relevance. Between 1960 and 1990, innumerable comparative studies of exercise testing and coronary angiography were published, providing exhaustive documentation of exercise testing as a diagnostic method, the gold standard being coronary angiography, which alone can diagnose significant stenosis. The test became more sensitive and more specific with the application of Bayes' theorem, which takes into account the prevalence of the disease and the patient's profile when interpreting results. Thereafter, ST-segment depression would no longer be read in the same way when recorded at 180 watts in a 40-year-old asymptomatic subject or at 60 watts in a 70-year-old angina patient.

At the same time, the number of indications for exercise testing increased. It was no longer taboo to test a patient with a recent myocardial infarction, which previously had been an absolute contraindication. At the end of the 1980s, it would even be considered useful, without danger, and of good prognostic value to give patients who suffered myocardial infarction an exercise test just before they left the hospital.

THE 1980s

THE 1980s SAW THE RISE OF CORONARY ANGIOPLASTY, WIDESPREAD USE OF EXERCISE TESTING, AND THE DEVELOPMENT OF COMPLEMENTARY TECHNIQUES. Exercise testing became a widely performed noninvasive cardiac examination, used for screening based on risk profile, follow-up after interventional cardiology or by-pass surgery, and assessment for rehabilitation programs. Its role was no longer merely diagnosis of coronary disease, but also and perhaps above all assessment of prognosis and of the risk of disease progression. Risk profiling has a major impact on therapeutic decisions, as some treatments involve a certain amount of risk to which, by definition, it is pointless to expose a low-risk patient. Combining exercise testing with isotopes helped refine diagnoses and assess the risk of progression, and so rationalize the indications for revascularization, for example.

This is the best known and traditional aspect of the test, but today exercise testing offers other possibilities and tomorrow it will offer even more, including analysis of expired gas, sharper assessment of disturbance of cellular energy balance with visualization of various segments of the myocardium using metabolic tracers combined with isotopes, assessment of LV function using ultrasound combined with exercise, quantification of functional capacities indicating degree of autonomy, noninvasive assessment of cardiac output during exercise, and more. The exercise test's multiple facets and the growing amount of information it can provide have increased its use as a means of exploring various aspects of the heart. In France, for example, a survey (outside the public sector) undertaken by the CNAM recorded 881 000 exercise tests carried out in 2006, including 121 000 combined with radionuclide imaging.

In 100 years of exploration of the heart's electrical activity, technical innovations and challenges to their clinical relevance have never ceased. This extraordinary story is far from over, and is still being written day after day.

Physiology –
Pathophysiology:

back
to basics

GENERAL CASES

Exercise testing (ET) is the most physiological method for testing a subject's physical capacities and limits. Dynamic exercise is the reference test, beginning with warm-up, followed by a steady increase to bring the subject to maximum effort in less than 20 minutes.

This is followed by a recovery period, which allows for a return to initial values. The muscles brought into play consume oxygen (O_2) and energy substrates, leading to changes in heart rate, blood pressure, respiration, and muscles.

CARDIAC RESPONSE

> **Cardiac output (Q) in liters per minute equals SV x HR where:**
> **SV is stroke volume (mL), ie, end-diastolic volume minus end-systolic volume, and HR is heart rate (beats per minute)**
> **SV: EDV-ESV.**
> **(EDV: end diastolic volume; ESV: end systolic volume)**

During exercise, cardiac output increases in two ways:
- Stroke volume (SV) increases to about 40% of maximum capacity, then plateaus;
- Heart rate (HR) increases linearly to maximum HR, with slight variations: during the initial phase of exercise, the immediate HR increase is due to a decrease in the influence of the parasympathetic nervous system, but also to activation of the sympathetic nervous system. The respective contribution of each system varies between subjects.

ET should avoid large load increments, which dissociate HR and oxygen uptake (VO_2).

The test should not exceed 20 minutes, because the rise in body temperature will produce partial blood redistribution due to increased HR.

VENTILATORY RESPONSE

> **Ventilation (VE) in liters per minute equals TV x RR where:**
> **TV is tidal volume (mL), the volume mobilized by each cycle, and RR is respiratory rate (breaths per minute)**

During exercise, ventilation increases in two ways:
- At the start of exercise, tidal volume (TV) increases to about 60% of peak oxygen uptake (VO_2 max);
- Respiratory rate (RR) initially increases slightly but by the end of exercise has risen considerably.

The maximum breathing capacity (MBC) is determined based on the theoretical maximum breathing capacity (35 or 40 FEV_1; FEV_1 = forced expiratory volume in one second).

Oxygenation can be approximated non-invasively using the degree of oxygen saturation in capillary blood, or it can be measured by arterial blood gas sampling (PpO_2 = partial pressure of oxygen).

PERIPHERAL RESPONSE

Arterial vasodilation in active muscles is related to a decrease in vascular resistance, with the mean blood pressure (MBP) rising slightly.

> **MBP = (SBP + 2 DBP)/3**
> **SBP = systolic blood pressure**
> **DBP = diastolic blood pressure**

SBP rises in proportion to exercise intensity; DBP remains essentially stable.

> **These data are linked to Q, as expressed in the equation**
> **Q = MBP/TPR** *(TPR = total peripheral resistance).*

The oxygen content in the arteries (CaO_2) and veins (CvO_2) is used to measure energy substrate and oxygen (O_2) delivery to active areas and their use by muscle fibers.

> **These data are linked to Q, as expressed in the equation**
> **Q = VO_2/(CaO_2 − CvO_2).**

MUSCLE RESPONSE

Two types of metabolism are activated during exercise testing:
- Aerobic metabolism (AM) is the preferred metabolism in humans and is very efficient, but requires oxygen. It is measured by oxygen uptake (VO_2), and its maximum value is referred to as VO_2 max;

- Anaerobic lactate metabolism (ALM) is less efficient, but does not require oxygen. It causes intra- and extracellular acidification. It is assessed based on blood bicarbonate and lactic acid levels.

As exercise intensity increases, so does anaerobic lactate metabolism, resulting in lactate and bicarbonate production and hyperventilation.

> **These are linked to Q, as expressed in the equation**
> $Q = VO_2/(CaO_2 - CvO_2)$.

These responses to exercise can be used to determine a subject's maximum capacity (W max or VO_2 max), which prognostic value is well documented.

RECOVERY
Changes in the various parameters can be observed during a recovery period of 5 to 6 minutes (active or passive, depending on the goals of the test).

TRAINED SUBJECTS
Exercise testing should be adapted (duration, initial load, increment duration) to subjects with higher capacities.

The target exercise level is 10% higher than usual norms (sex, age, weight) for 2 hours of weekly training, 20% for 4 hours/week, etc.

The highest level corresponds to more than 10 hours of training per week carried out at more than 60% of W max (or VO_2 max).

If there is no disease, the various systems function at full capacity and subjects can then be limited by various factors - muscle fatigue, polypnea, or general fatigue.

The nervous system plays an important role in trained subjects: major sympathetic stimulation, with the release of large amounts of adrenaline, increases exercise tolerance. The results then differ from the "norm":
- Maximum HR is variable, often higher than the theoretical maximum; HR decreases rapidly during recovery;
- SV rises with increase in EDV and in myocardial contractility;
- MBC is high, exceeding the theoretical MBC (40 FEV₁ in physically active subjects) due to an increase in TV max;

- Maximum systolic blood pressure is often higher than the usual values (adrenergic peak) and diastolic blood pressure is quite variable;
- Better oxygen diffusion in muscle capillaries causes the difference between arterial and venous oxygen uptake (CaO_2 - CvO_2) to rise;
- Blood lactate levels are high immediately after exercise and during early recovery;
- VO_2 max and W max increase.

In order to consider these cardiocirculatory and ventilatory responses as "unusual", the subject has to tolerate the test perfectly and recover rapidly.

CORONARY PATIENTS

In patients with coronary disease that limits oxygen delivery to myocardial cells, a discrepancy between supply and demand can be observed during exercise. Myocardial demand for O_2 (MVO_2) and for energy substrates rises during exercise due to increased HR, intraventricular and intraparietal pressure, myocardial contractility and blood pressure (STT = HR x SBP) (STT = systolic tension time or double product).

A normal increase of coronary blood flow during exercise can be disrupted in cases of significant coronary stenosis (ie, stenosis that does not allow the normal 4- to 5-fold increase [from baseline] in coronary blood flow during exercise).

Stenosis that reduces the luminal diameter by 50% to 80% allows some increase in coronary blood flow during exercise, but not enough to meet the increased demand. Stenosis that reduces the luminal diameter by 80% to 90% prevents any increase in coronary blood flow during exercise, so that flow remains stable despite the increased demand, thus generating ischemia.

A 90% reduction may decrease absolute coronary blood flow during exercise. When the stenosis is tight, the distal coronary arteries dilate considerably to maintain the resting blood flow. This distal vasodilation results in a loss of energy (loss of pressure) downstream from the stenosis. Any further stimulus (exercise, emotional response, etc.) that increases energy loss can cause a sharp drop in coronary blood flow.

Their vasomotor properties enable coronary vessels, like all other vessels, to vary in diameter by ± 30%, and sometimes much more. The endothelium plays a key role in this. In the normal subject, the (healthy) endothelium generates coronary vasodilation during exercise, which is said to be flow-dependent: flow increase causes vasodilation (mediator = nitric oxide or NO). Endothelial dysfunction can lead to coronary vasoconstriction during exercise (for example, increasing stenosis from 40% to 60%).

The coronary endothelium is very sensitive to environmental conditions, such as smoking, diabetes, high blood pressure, dyslipidemia, inflammation, sympathetic/parasympathetic balance, etc.

An imbalance between supply and demand is described as myocardial ischemia.

Myocardial ischemia has a number of consequences:
- **Mechanical:** decreased SV, following decreases in systolic contractility and EDV (quick filling phase via impaired active relaxation);
- **Electrical:** changes in repolarization and arrhythmia following electrophysiological and ionic disturbances (defective sodium and potassium pumps, metabolic acidosis);
- **Clinical:** intermittent chest pain of variable intensity generated by stimulation of sympathetic nerve endings (eighth cervical root and first four dorsal roots). When ischemia is very great, poor pressure adaptation due to severe left ventricular dysfunction can be observed;
- **Functional:** reduced W max (or VO_2 max) due to decreased perfusion in peripheral muscles (prognostic value).

Some authors suggest performing a "sharp" sensitization test after recovery from the traditional test, at an intensity close to W max.

Many cardiovascular drugs interfere with cardiovascular adaptation and so alter the conditions under which ischemia occurs. The timing of medication intake should then be noted (pharmacokinetics).

PATIENTS WITH HEART FAILURE

Heart failure is characterized by changes in the heart's "pumping" function, notably a decrease in the volume of blood ejected by the left ventricle at each systole. Blood accumulates upstream (lungs) and downstream flow diminishes (muscles, digestive organs). Efficient self-regulatory systems protect the brain and kidneys to some extent: their blood flow remains stable despite decreased perfusion pressure. Cardiac (increased HR and EDV) and peripheral compensatory mechanisms come into play, and arterial vasoconstriction seeks to maintain optimal organ perfusion pressure.

The effects of heart failure on the various systems depend on its severity and duration, and on what treatment is initiated.

Exercise testing combined with expired gas analysis can be used to study not only cardiac function, but also ventilation and energy metabolism.

HEART

> **HR: tachycardia at rest and during exercise.**
> **SV: The VO_2/HR relationship is used to assess how SV changes during exercise;**
> **this is often called the oxygen pulse and is equal to**
> **SV x (CaO_2 - CvO_2). In heart disease, CaO_2 - CvO_2 does not change.**

Blood pressure profile during exercise indicates the efficiency of the heart pump. Depending on how severe the heart failure is, systolic pressure (SBP) can increase slightly (less than 20 mm Hg), remain stable, or even decrease during exercise.

Blood pressure patterns during exercise are of high prognostic value in heart failure.

LUNGS

Fluid in the various parts of the lungs results in:
- Decreased vital capacity (VC) and bronchial and pulmonary compliance;
- Decreased TV max due to restriction;
- Increased respiratory rate;
- Dynamic hyperinflation due to obstruction;
- Increased respiratory equivalents in CO_2 (VE/VCO_2) and O_2 (VE/VO_2).

VE/VCO_2 has high prognostic value.

MUSCLES

The decrease in muscle perfusion resulting from decreased cardiac output (Q) and increased peripheral resistance (sympathetic vasoconstriction) causes muscles to favor low-efficiency anaerobic metabolism, which leads to early intra- and extracellular acidification. The consequences are:

- Less strength corresponding to the anaerobic threshold, expressed in watts or in metabolic equivalents (METs); anaerobic threshold defines what the subject can do without discomfort, or in other words, his or her degree of autonomy;

The anaerobic threshold has prognostic value.

- Lower maximum aerobic capacities, with no plateau of myocardial oxygen consumption (VO_2 max), the maximum value of VO_2 at rest being called peak VO_2.

Peak VO_2 has prognostic value.

HYPERTENSIVE PATIENTS

High peripheral resistance at rest and during exercise accompanies essential hypertension. Blood pressure is higher, and the systolic blood pressure slope parallels that in normotensive subjects, or may be steeper, depending on the severity of hypertension. Diastolic blood pressure will depend on how peripheral resistance changes during exercise. The test should be interrupted if systolic blood pressure is >250 mm Hg or diastolic blood pressure is >130 mm Hg or both.

There is a slight increase in cardiac output, due to a decrease in maximum HR and maximum SV, resulting from changes in diastolic function (EDV). In the heart, there is a decrease in coronary reserve (peak flow/resting flow for a given perfusion pressure), resulting from numerous abnormalities, including thickening of the arteriolar wall, endothelial dysfunction, change in vasomotricity, and sympathetic hyperactivity.

Capillary density is reduced in severe myocardial hypertrophy. In the myocardium, a rise in left ventricular end-diastolic pressure could result in inadequate perfusion of the subendocardial layers. All these disorders could result in authentic, exercise-induced myocardial ischemia that is not linked to stenoses in large coronary vessels. At the periphery, excessive arterial vasoconstriction reduces blood supply to active muscles, which is reflected by lower aerobic capacities (VO_2 max) than in normotensive subjects.

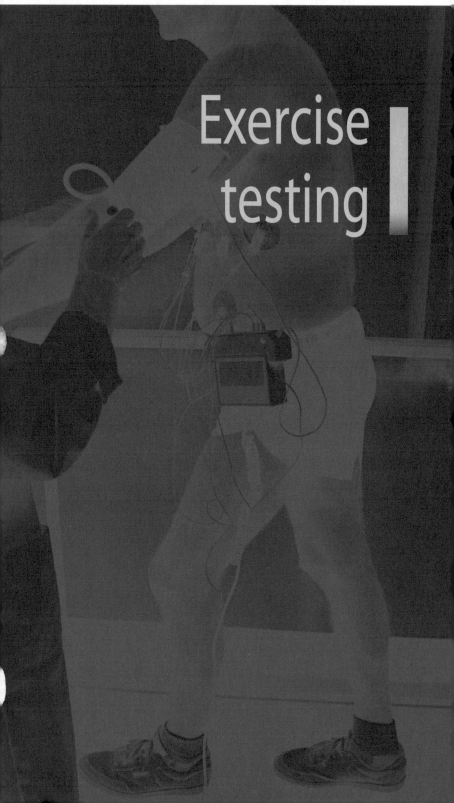

Exercise testing

INTRODUCTION

Exercise testing is simple, noninvasive, easily available, and inexpensive. It is a physiological test that reproduces a common human action. Considering these advantages, the information exercise testing provides, both for the diagnosis and prognosis of heart disease, is remarkable. It is an irreplaceable aid for the clinical management of coronary artery disease, both at the initial stage and during follow-up.

FACILITIES, STAFF AND EQUIPMENT

FACILITIES

Exercise testing requires appropriate conditions:

▶ A spacious room, aerated or if possible ventilated, at a temperature around 20°C;

▶ An examination bed for lying the patient down if necessary;

▶ Resuscitation equipment (regularly checked and updated resuscitation trolley), with at least: intubation and ventilation equipment, defibrillator, drugs (sodium bicarbonate, 5% glucose, nitrate derivatives, injectable or oral antiarrhythmic agents-lidocaine, β-blockers, adenosine triphosphate, adrenergic products such as isoprenaline, adrenaline, atropine sulfate, injectable furosemide), oxygen supply;

▶ The facilities should be located near an intensive care unit.

STAFF

The examining cardiologist should be thoroughly familiar with exercise testing. Though there are no standards in the matter, one can consider 20 exercise tests a month as a minimum. The cardiologist should be assisted by a nurse with adequate training and familiarity with the test.

EQUIPMENT

▶ **A cycle ergometer is commonly used in Europe;** it is economical and makes less noise than the treadmill, and there are fewer artifacts in the tracings. The maximum predicted heart rate (HR) is more difficult to reach, while the so-called double product (HR times systolic blood pressure) is more or less equivalent for the two methods, as the rise in blood pressure is greater on a bicycle (Table I).

▶ **The treadmill is widely used in the United States;** walking is more physiological and easier (some people do not know how to pedal). The maximum predicted HR is more easily reached; oxygen uptake (VO_2 max) is higher than that obtained on a cycle ergometer (larger muscle groups are involved).

Table I - Treadmill or cycle ergometer?		
	Treadmill	**Cycle ergometer**
Preferential use	United States	Europe
Price	High	Moderate
Bulk, noise	High	Moderate
BP measurement	Sometimes difficult	Easy
ECG artifacts	Frequent	Less frequent
Reaching MPHR	Easy	More difficult
Test feasibility	Optimal (everyone can walk)	Some people cannot pedal

EXERCISE TESTING PROCEDURE

CHECK FOR ABSENCE OF CONTRAINDICATIONS

Absolute contraindications: persistent thoracic pain, especially if associated with a modification of the original ECG, tight aortic stenosis, recent myocardial infarction (3 to 5 days), unstable angina, tight stenosis of the left main coronary artery, severe, uncontrolled arrhythmia, congestive heart failure, pulmonary embolism, peripheral thrombosis, myocarditis, pericarditis or endocarditis, intraventricular thrombus, aortic dissection, or patient incapacity or refusal.

Relative contraindications: moderate aortic stenosis, uncontrolled hypertension, electrolytic abnormalities, severe hypertrophic cardio-myopathy, significant hypertrophic obstructive cardiomyopathy, uncooperative patient, high-degree atrioventricular block, progressive general diseases, co-morbidities, short life expectancy (Table II).

Table II - Exercise test contraindications	
Absolute	**Relative**
Persistent chest pain associated with ECG modification	Moderate aortic stenosis
Tight aortic stenosis	Uncontrolled high BP
Very recent myocardial infarction or unstable angina	Abnormal serum potassium
Uncontrolled arrhythmia or congestive heart failure	Severe hypertrophic cardiomyopathy
Progressive myocarditis, pericarditis, or endocarditis	Moderate-degree aortic valve stenosis
Aortic dissection	Lack of patient cooperation
Patient refusal or incapacity	Comorbidities, reduced life expectancy

ASSESS THE RELEVANCE OF THE INDICATION
Briefly, the lower the probability of coronary disease, the higher the risk of false positives; this is particularly true in women under the age of 60. In addition, three specific situations should be mentioned. LBBB, WPW, and pacemakers make ST segment interpretation impossible. Other tests are needed to identify ischemia. Yet, stress testing can effectively detect rhythm troubles and assess physical capacity. Finally, stress testing value is reduced after an infarction or in the presence of marked EKG alterations at rest, or in patients receiving anti-arrhythmic treatments such as digitalis.

PERFORM A QUICK CLINICAL EXAMINATION
Patent signs of congestive heart failure and aortic or carotid stenosis should be ruled out.

MAKE SURE THE PATIENT UNDERSTANDS THE PROCEDURE
Ensure that the subject has properly understood the nature of the test and its goal, and is appropriately dressed. Gather information about current treatments and examine the doctor's prescription. Have the patient sign the informed consent form (*see sidebar*).

PREPARE THE SKIN, POSITION THE BLOOD PRESSURE CUFF
Abrasion of the skin improves signal quality and is essential to prevent artifacts, which can lead to misinterpretation.

CHOOSE THE EXERCISE PROTOCOL
The test **has to be adapted** so the patient reaches maximum exercise intensity in about 10 minutes. The test will generally last 8 to 12 minutes for an "average" subject, and longer for trained subjects. A single protocol cannot be applied to different patients.

▶ **Treadmill:** The Bruce protocol allows for 3-minute stages and is well adapted to male subjects in their fifties; it is often useful for athletes to allow for a higher increment, while a more progressive increment is used for elderly, sedentary, or weary subjects.

▶ **Cycle ergometer:** Conventionally, 30 W every 3 minutes. Maximum exercise intensity can be reached more easily with a ramped protocol: using the calculated theoretical maximum exercise intensity (Table III), 20% load for first 2 minutes, then 10%/minute increments to reach maximum intensity in 10 minutes.

Table III - Predicted target exercise intensity								
Height / Age	150	155	160	165	170	175	180	185	190
30	172	182	192	202	212	222	232	242	252
35	160	170	180	190	200	210	220	230	240
40	148	158	168	178	188	198	208	218	228
45	137	147	157	167	177	187	197	207	217
50	125	135	145	155	165	175	185	195	205
55	113	123	133	143	153	163	173	183	193
60	101	111	121	131	141	151	161	171	181
65	89	99	109	119	129	139	149	159	169
70	77	87	97	107	117	127	137	147	157
75	65	75	85	95	105	115	125	135	145
80	53	63	73	83	93	103	113	123	133
85	41	51	61	71	81	91	101	111	121

* For women intensity should be 80 % of the figure indicated

EXAMPLE OF INFORMED CONSENT FORM

Why are you having an exercise test?

Exercise electrocardiography will be performed to help detect, diagnose, and evaluate a cardiovascular problem.

What happens during the test?

You are going to exercise on a cycle ergometer or a treadmill for a few minutes. During the test, the electrical activity of your heart (electrocardiogram) and your blood pressure will be monitored continuously, in order to detect any possible abnormalities. This test requires your active participation because, for it to be useful, you have to reach a sufficient exercise intensity to ensure an appropriate increase in heart rate.

Are there any risks?

The laboratory where the test is performed is run by skilled and experienced staff. It is equipped with all the devices and equipment needed to optimize safety and minimize risk. Complications are therefore exceptional. It is important to understand that the risk incurred because of an undetected heart problem is greater than the risk associated with exercise testing.

What are the advantages of exercise testing?

It screens for problems that cannot be detected at rest and that only come to light with exercise. The results will be sent to your doctor, who will prescribe any treatment you may need, or further tests. This document is not a discharge of responsibility, and our team is available should you require further information.

I acknowledge that the nature of exercise testing, its risks and advantages have been explained to me in terms that I understand and that all the questions I have asked have been satisfactorily answered.

Patient's signature: **Doctor's signature:**

MONITORING DURING EXERCISE TESTING

Monitoring should cover:

- Clinical signs: Chest pain? Dyspnea? Skin color?
- Electrocardiographic signs: increase in HR with exercise, arrhythmia, ST-segment elevation or depression, etc. Monitoring should be constant throughout the test. Most electrocardiographic devices are generally 12-lead and provide a printout on request;
- Manometric signs: blood pressure is measured at the beginning and at each exercise level, to note whether its increase is normal, excessive, or insufficient.

The criteria for interrupting the test (Table IV) are as follows:

▶ *Absolute:*

- Drop in blood pressure, signs of low output (paleness, cold skin, cyanosis);
- Severe angina, ST-segment elevation;
- Severe ventricular arrhythmia or conduction disorder;
- Patient request;
- Technical problem (BP or ECG monitoring failure).

▶ *Relative:*

- Moderate angina, fatigue or dyspnea, claudication, marked ST-segment depression;
- BP 250/115 mm Hg;
- Uncontrolled ventricular extrasystoles, supraventricular tachycardia.

Table IV - Reasons for stopping exercise testing	
Absolute	**Relative**
Drop in blood pressure	ST-segment depression > 2 mm
ST-segment elevation	Fatigue, dyspnea, moderate angina, claudication
Severe angina, severe arrhythmia	High blood pressure, arrhythmia
Patient refusal	Uncooperative patient

▶ *Otherwise, the test is interrupted when:*
  • Theoretical maximum exercise intensity is reached;
  • Theoretical maximum HR is reached (HRmax = 220 – age).
These figures are a guide and do not mandate interruption of testing.

Once exercise has ceased, monitoring should continue until ECG parameters, HR, and blood pressure return to baseline. If vasovagal syncope occurs, one should position the patient supine and take appropriate measures (raise legs, administer atropine, etc.).

WHAT ARE THE RISKS OF EXERCISE TESTING?
Average risks documented in hundreds of thousands of subjects are easily understood (Table V), but in fact risk varies greatly depending on the subjects: almost nil for young subjects with no specific medical history, it can become significant for an elderly patient with heart disease or other comorbidities (renal failure, cancer, etc).

Table V - Risks associated with exercise testing	
Risk	**Mean frequency**
Vasovagal episode	3 to 5%
Severe arrhythmia	1/20 000
Myocardial infarction	1/50 000
Death	1/70 000

INTERPRETING EXERCISE TESTING
FUNCTIONAL CAPACITY
It can be expressed by the:
  • Level of exercise achieved (expressed in watts on a cycle ergometer);
  • Double product, ie, systolic blood pressure x HR, measured at maximum exercise intensity;
  • Maximum HR reached relative to the target HR;
  • Duration of the exercise.
The maximum oxygen uptake, or VO_2 max, is maximum cardiac output multiplied by the arteriovenous difference in oxygen content. It is an excellent indication of physical capacity, and in a normal sedentary adult is between 2.5 and 4.5 ml O_2/kg/min, and decreases with age.

Functional capacity (level of exercise performed) is an important and independent predictive factor for cardiovascular and overall mortality, in both symptomatic subjects and patients with coronary artery disease. Ability to reach an exercise intensity above 10 metabolic equivalents (METs) indicates an excellent prognosis even in the presence of coronary heart disease. On the contrary, subjects unable to reach 5 METs have a mortality risk twice that of subjects whose physical capacity is higher than or equal to 8 METs. For each additional MET performed, the risk of dying decreases by 10% to 15%.

The predictive value of functional capacity is comparable to that of scintigraphic defects and higher than that of the severity of coronary lesions, or ST-segment depression (Table VI).

Table VI - METs/watts equivalence	
Watts	**METs**
250	13/14
225	12
200	11
175	9/10
150	8
125	7
100	6
75	5
50	3/4
25	2/3

METs: *metabolic equivalents.*

HEART RATE

HR rate is a key parameter in exercise testing, and at rest is of prognostic value: the higher the HR, the greater the risk of a cardiovascular incident. The maximum HR during exercise depends on age, level of training, type of exercise, presence or not of cardiopathy, and the patient's motivation. The target is the predicted maximum, which is 220 minus the subject's age.

The parameters most commonly used to analyze HR during exercise testing are:

- The percentage of predicted maximum HR reached: for example, if a 62-year-old subject reaches a maximum HR of 127 beats per minute (bpm), with an MPHR of: 220 − 62 = 158 bpm, this subject performed 127/158 = 80% of his MPHR;
- Cardiac reserve, which is the difference between the MPHR and HR at rest;
- Chronotropic reserve, which is the MPHR reached - HR at rest/cardiac reserve. For example, if a subject has a MPHR of 166 bpm, a HR of 60 bpm at rest and reaches a HR of 155 bpm, his chronotropic reserve is 155 − 60/166 − 60 = 89%. Less than 80% indicates chronotropic incompetence, which is a poor prognostic criterion independent of age and functional capacity.

Many recent studies have shown a significant link between mortality and HR recovery (HRR), which is the difference between maximum HR during exercise and HR after one minute of recovery. Of mean value 17 bpm, HRR is considered abnormal when below 12 bpm, and is independent of studied groups and treatment (Table VII).

Table VII - Heart rate: a key parameter of exercise testing		
HR at rest	Normal between 50 and 70 bpm	Poorer prognosis if high
MPHR (maximum predicted heart rate)	220 - age	Submaximal if < 85% of MPHR
Chronotropic reserve	Max HR - HR at rest/ MPHR - HR at rest	Unfavorable prognosis if < 80% of the predicted value
Recovery HR	Slowing down of HR after one minute of recovery	Unfavorable prognosis if < 12 bpm

Symptoms
During testing, dyspnea (physiological or not), typical or atypical chest pain, general fatigue, muscle fatigue in lower limbs, other symptoms (vertigo, headache, etc.) should be noted.

ST-segment depression: a classic sign of ischemia
ST-segment depression, the commonest manifestation of exercise-induced ischemia, reflects subendocardial hypoperfusion, but does not have any localization value. It is said to be significant when it is horizontal (or downsloping), measures more than one millimeter 80 ms after the J point, and concords in several leads. The reliability of "averaged" recordings is imperfect, so it is essential to make sure that the ST-segment depression on the original recording is genuine. This underlines the importance of proper signal collection, which depends on adequate skin preparation.

The final interpretation of ST-segment depression depends on the clinical context: it predictably corresponds to significant myocardial ischemia if recorded at low exercise intensity in a 72-year-old man, who simultaneously describes chest pain. But the same ST segment depression has every chance of being a "false positive" if recorded at maximum exercise intensity in a 52-year-old woman with mitral valve prolapse. More generally, interpretation of repolarization takes into consideration age, sex, associated functional signs, the number of leads concerned by the ST-segment depression, the exercise intensity at which depression occurred and its amplitude, and the speed of its normalization during recovery. The lower the pre-test probability, the greater the risk of false positives. It is therefore important to evaluate pre-test probability. The test is especially useful if this probability is intermediate; if pre-test probability is very high or very low, the diagnosis is essentially clinical.

To be of diagnostic value, the ST-segment depression should be:
- *at least 1 mm;*
- *80 ms after the J point;*
- *in two concordant leads;*
- *horizontal or downsloping.*

It has even more value if it:
- *persists or worsens during recovery;*
- *is accompanied by chest pain or by arrhythmia, especially ventricular.*

It may be a false positive in the following cases:
- *drug administration (amiodarone, digitalis derivatives, etc.);*
- *high blood pressure, left ventricular hypertrophy;*
- *young, asymptomatic subject;*
- *mitral valve prolapse.*

Abnormal repolarization at rest

LBBB, Wolff-Parkinson-White syndrome, and electrotrained rhythm prevent ST analysis during exercise, and other tests are required to screen for ischemia. However, exercise testing can be performed to screen for rhythmic disorders, monitor a pacemaker, or evaluate functional capacity.

More generally, test reliability is lower when repolarization abnormalities of any kind are present initially. In principle, it is reassuring if they disappear during exercise, but no firm conclusion can be drawn should they persist or worsen, and further testing may be required.

Remarks

1 - Coronary artery disease (in the sense of proximal coronary stenosis) is not the only cause of ST-segment depression during exercise: myocardial hypertrophy, resulting from high blood pressure for example, and some myocardiopathies as well as some drug treatments can induce authentic depressions not corresponding to the presence of "significant" coronary stenosis.

2 - Atrial repolarization can sometimes mimic an authentic depression (sum of p plus T). This phenomenon is all the more common when there is atrial hypertrophy, such as in high blood pressure or congestive heart failure.

3 - ST-segment analysis can be refined by other criteria:
- Taking into consideration HR in the evaluation of ST-segment depression is always useful: the nonsignificant nature of ST-segment depression of 0.5 mm could be reconsidered if it occurs for an increase in HR of 15 bpm; it could be equal to a depression of 1 mm obtained after an HR increase of 30 bpm. The slope of the relation ST-segment depression vs HR can be very useful in interpreting exercise testing.
- Change in ST-segment depression during recovery is also informative: a depression that resolves quickly during recovery is more suggestive of a false positive than a depression that persists or more particularly that rises during recovery.
- Widening QRS is a sign of ischemia, albeit minor compared with repolarization modifications. The disappearance of the Q wave in V5 during exercise is pathognomonic of ischemia.

ST-segment elevation

ST-segment elevation during exercise is not exceptional, but requires special attention. ST-segment elevation is common when there are sequelae of necrosis, and normally reflects a dyskinetic zone. But in the absence of myocardial infarction, ST-segment elevation corresponds to severe, transmural ischemia with good localization value.

It may be associated with a mirror image ST-segment depression and is an emergency, requiring rapid hospitalization and coronary angiography. Left main coronary stenosis or three-vessel disease is not exceptional in these cases.

Hazards requiring immediate attention during exercise testing:

- *ST-segment elevation during exercise, especially if associated with chest pain;*
- *Blood pressure drop during exercise, ventricular tachycardia during exercise;*
- *ST-segment depression that does not resolve during recovery.*

OTHER SIGNS

The occurrence of RBBB or LBBB during exercise is most often of degenerative origin. If the conductive disorder is preceded by anginal pain or ST-segment depression or both - or is noted early typically below 120 bpm - it is probably of ischemic origin. As a general rule, the occurrence of LBBB during exercise is a good indication for radionuclide imaging and may avoid pointless coronary angiography.
The occurrence of a left anterior hemiblock during exercise is very commonly associated with proximal stenosis of the anterior descending coronary artery.

Ventricular arrhythmia triggered by exercise has no formal diagnostic value, but suggests underlying heart disease, which may or may not be ischemic. Prognosis is worse if it occurs during recovery. The disappearance of extrasystoles (present at rest) during exercise suggests they are harmless.

TYPICAL EXERCISE TESTING REPORT

Prescribing physician:

Patient's name:
Date of birth / Sex / Height/ Weight:
Address:

Reasons for the test, clinical context:
- Functional signs (typical, suspect, atypical, absent);
- Medical history (revascularization, myocardial infarction, etc.);
- Current treatment (especially β-blockers);
- Risk factors.

Protocol:
- Cycle ergometer or treadmill, protocol used;
- Target heart rate, target exercise level.

Results:
- Initial state: ECG, HR, BP;
- Reasons for stopping the exercise (fatigue, dyspnea, chest pain, maximum predicted exercise intensity or HR reached, other);
- Percentage of maximum predicted achieved (exercise intensity and HR);
- ECG during exercise: ST segment, QRS changes, T wave, arrhythmia;
- BP profile during exercise;
- Recovery: clinical or ECG abnormality.

CONCLUSION

Classify the test as:
- Negative (normal);
- Positive, in this case, specify the possible presence of severity criteria
- Or borderline (submaximal, ascending ST-depression, abnormal initial ECG, etc.).

CLINICAL VALUE OF EXERCISE TESTING

COMPARISON WITH CORONARY ANGIOGRAPHY

Historically, exercise testing had been widely compared with coronary angiography, the gold standard for coronary artery disease. These comparisons have been the subject of numerous publications, with results noticeably varying from one study to another, depending on the prevalence of coronary disease among the studied population, the technique used for exercise testing, and the criteria of "significant" stenosis (50% or 70% reduction in luminal diameter).

In terms of its diagnostic value, it is generally agreed that, in an unselected population, exercise testing has a sensitivity, specificity, positive predictive value, and negative predictive value of around 70%,. These numbers improve greatly in a population where the prevalence of coronary disease is high, or when the expertise of the center performing the exercise testing is high.

PROGNOSTIC VALUE OF EXERCISE TESTING

With the extensive development of percutaneous revascularization techniques, it has become necessary to combine diagnostic information (Is there a significant coronary stenosis?) with prognostic information (What is the risk for the patient?). The anatomy of a stenosis does not necessarily allow for a precise evaluation of the risk.

Because the risk of angioplasty and stenting is not nil (1% to 2% for the procedure itself, plus the risks linked to restenosis and antiplatelet/anticoagulant drugs), it is important to identify patients at sufficiently high risk to justify treatment with non-negligible short-, medium-, and long-term iatrogenic effects.

The prognostic value of exercise testing is supported by numerous studies concerning thousands of patients: in the short term, ST-segment elevation during exercise and large ST-segment depression associated with a drop in blood pressure are serious signs requiring immediate action. In the medium or long term, physical capacity, HR during exercise and its rate of normalization during recovery are parameters of high prognostic value.

WHAT SHOULD BE DONE WITH EXERCISE TEST RESULTS?

3 situations can be identified:

The exercise test is clearly positive

Basically, there are three levels of risk, corresponding to three distinct practical approaches.

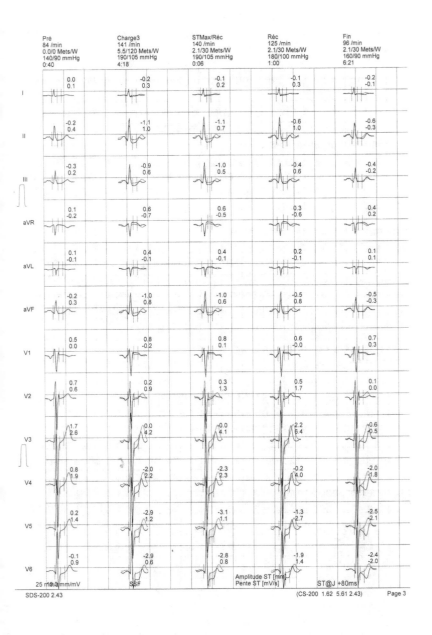

Fig. 1 - Positive exercise testing.

▶ *Very high risk:* ST-segment elevation during exercise (apart from a myocardial infarction scar), or ST-segment depression greater than 2 mm associated with blood pressure drop, or simple positive findings that do not change at the end of the exercise in spite of several minutes of recovery: this indicates the need for an emergency coronary angiography.

▶ *Significant risk:* Clear ST-segment depression in several leads, associated with chest pain at a submaximal exercise intensity: indication for coronary angiography.

▶ *Moderate but significant risk:* Positive electrocardiographic findings without clinical severity criteria, good physical performance: indication to complete the risk assessment (calcium scoring, myocardial SPECT).

Exercise test is clearly negative

The exercise intensity and HR reached are normal with regard to age, and there are no suspicious electrocardiographic abnormalities: simple clinical supervision is most often recommended. If the good result of the exercise testing contradicts the clinical context (angina, age, risk factors), further exploration is legitimate because the probability of a false negative is 20% in an intermediate risk population.

Exercise test findings are borderline

Test findings are borderline if the exercise intensity and HR reached are submaximal or there is ascending ST-segment depression (relative to theoretical maximum HR or expected exercise intensity) or the findings are clinically positive with no associated electrocardiographic abnormality or are positive only during recovery or are difficult to interpret because some abnormalities are present on the ECG at rest: myocardial infarction scar, repolarization disorders, LVH, LBBB, Wolff-Parkinson-White syndrome, etc. Borderline exercise test findings are a good indication for radionuclide myocardial perfusion imaging or, if the probability of coronary disease is very low (low prevalence), for multidetector computed tomography (Table VIII).

Table VIII - What is a borderline exercise test?
• Submaximal exercise test;
• Ascending ST-segment depression;
• ST-segment depression only during recovery;
• Test clinically positive, with no ECG abnormalities;
• Repolarization abnormalities present at rest: myocardial infarction scar, LBBB, RBBB, Wolff-Parkinson-White syndrome, pacemaker, left ventricular hypertrophy.

GENERAL INDICATIONS FOR EXERCISE TESTING
DIAGNOSIS OF CORONARY ARTERY DISEASE

Diagnosis of coronary artery disease is the main indication for exercise testing, considering symptoms typically classified into three groups (Table IX):

▶ Typical angina: Retrosternal constrictive pain, crushing, vice-like, sometimes irradiating in the jaws and arms, indicated by the palm of the hand, triggered by exercise, especially walking on a slope or in cold weather, alleviated by the end of exercise, eased by nitrates;

▶ Atypical chest pain: Thoracic pain or discomfort that can have some but not all of the characteristics of typical angina. Atypical chest pain is one of the best indications for exercise testing;

▶ Non-coronary chest pain: Tingling, dorsalgia, epigastralgia, etc. In principle, these symptoms are not very suggestive and their analysis should be combined with clinical data (especially age and sex) but, in some rare cases, they can mask authentic coronary disease. More recently, unexplained dyspnea of recent occurrence has been identified as a suspicious functional sign, requiring investigation for coronary insufficiency.

Table IX - Major indications for exercise testing	
Indications	**Comments**
Diagnosis of chest pain or dyspnea	The diagnostic value of exercise testing depends on the characteristics of chest pain, age, sex, and the extent of ST-segment depression.
Asymptomatic subject	Exercise testing is justified if there are several risk factors, a high-risk profession, or an athletic activity.
After revascularization or myocardial infarction	Exercise testing alone is of limited value. Combine with isotopic techniques.
Women	False positives are frequent.
Elderly subjects	Protocol must be adapted. High prevalence of coronary disease.
Trained subjects	Protocol must be adapted. Frequent repolarization disorders. Value of complementary techniques (echocardiography, isotopes, computed tomography).

In practice:
- When there is low probability of coronary disease (young subject, asymptomatic or few symptoms), exercise test findings are often normal and therefore have a strong negative predictive value, which is reassuring. Positive tests are rarer and are frequently false positives. These situations can be clarified by myocardial perfusion imaging;
- When there is an intermediate probability of coronary disease, stress testing is specifically indicated with a good positive predictive value. Yet, the negative predictive value of exercise testing is imperfect, since authentic coronary disease can be present in about 2/10 patients with normal exercise test findings. It may be interesting to combine exercise testing and myocardial perfusion imaging;
- When there is a high probability of coronary disease (risk factors, typical angina), positive predictive value is high, and stress testing mainly has prognostic value. Yet, its negative predictive value is low: the number of patients with a false negative result is high.

EVALUATION OF KNOWN CORONARY ARTERY DISEASE
Exercise testing is often indicated to monitor coronary artery disease.

Efficacy of drug treatment
Drug efficacy is assessed in terms of improved functional capacity and elevation of the ischemic/anginal threshold. The test especially indicates the intensity of exercise the patient can safely perform below the ischemic threshold, given the well-known advantages of regular physical activity.

After angioplasty
Exercise testing (after the 15th day) can be used to check the procedure's effectiveness, and to guide rehabilitation followed by the return to work and to physical activity. It can be psychologically beneficial by reassuring the patient and his family. However, it should be noted that test sensitivity and specificity are lower after revascularization and imaging is frequently used to diagnose restenosis. Apart from classic signs, a reduction in functional capacity heralds possible restenosis (normally screened for between the third and sixth month).

After coronary by-pass surgery
In cases of postoperative chest pain, the test differentiates between ischemic and parietal pain, but the frequent presence of repolarization abnormalities at rest sometimes renders interpretation difficult. In the longer term, exercise testing detects recurrence of ischemia, whether linked to stenosis of a graft or to disease progression in another vessel.

Imaging is frequently required to localize and monitor the spread of ischemia. Exercise testing can be used to guide rehabilitation and the return to work and physical activity. Here again, it can be psychologically beneficial by reassuring the patient and his family.

After myocardial infarction

Here exercise testing is mainly of functional and prognostic value. A submaximal test from the fifth day and/or a symptom-limited test after 14 days may be needed to recommend physical activity, achieve rehabilitation, assess the prognosis, evaluate and adapt medical treatment, and allow the patient to leave the hospital and return to work.

The search for residual ischemia requires myocardial SPECT, because exercise testing is not sensitive or specific enough (the absence of ST-segment depression does not eliminate ischemia, its presence does not necessarily indicate it, and may be a "mirror" of the infarction).

SPECIFIC SITUATIONS

Woman

The risk of false positives is high, considering the classically low prevalence of coronary artery disease before the menopause. Resorting to radionuclide imaging or multidetector computed tomography is common when the probability of coronary disease is low.

Diabetes

Silent ischemia is frequent, but exercise testing should be targeted. Type 2 diabetic patients should be over the age of 60 or with known disease for more than 10 years, if there are two other associated risk factors. In type 1 diabetic patients, the criteria to look for are: age over 45, diabetes treated for more than 15 years, and presence of at least two other risk factors. In type 1 or 2 diabetic patients, the search for silent ischemia is justified once there is peripheral vascular impairment or proteinuria, whatever the age, or in the case of microalbuminuria in the presence of two other risk factors, or in the case of return to a sporting activity after the age of 45.

Asymptomatic subjects

The prevalence of coronary disease is low and systematic exercise testing should be reserved for subjects:
- With several risk factors;
- With peripheral vascular disease (legs, carotids);
- With a high-risk profession (airline pilot, public transport staff);
- Who wish to return to a physical activity/sport.

Elderly subjects
As the population ages, exercise testing and its indications are becoming more frequent in elderly patients, who increasingly wish to be physically active and do sport. The prevalence of disease is high and so is the positive predictive value. Comorbidity is common—cardiovascular disease (high blood pressure, conduction disorders, atrial fibrillation) and joint disorders—and so there is a need for adapted protocols, using small load increments when necessary.
Exercise testing can reveal ischemic abnormalities, but also arrhythmias or conduction disorders.

Trained subjects
Protocols need to be adapted to enable the test subject to reach maximum exercise intensity. Repolarization abnormalities are frequent, leading to difficulties in test interpretation, in subjects who are usually asymptomatic, which explains why radionuclide imaging is frequently used, or multidetector computed tomography if the prevalence is low.

Preoperative risk assessment for noncardiac surgery
Exercise testing is indicated in cases of major surgery, when there are risk factors, and especially if there is ischemic heart disease. Functional capacity is essential prognostically and theoretically and enables the assessment of surgical risk. In practice, however, a good standard test can rarely be performed in this population and so it is frequently necessary to resort to imaging with pharmacological stimulation.
In preoperative risk assessment, current international recommendations advocate that exercise testing or other functional tests should be performed according to the clinical situation, independently of surgery. One should do what would have been done if no surgery had been scheduled.

Congestive heart failure
Exercise testing is an essential tool for congestive heart failure, and is frequently associated with gas exchange measurements (VO_2; see specific chapter). Peak VO_2 is important because it is an independent marker of the prognosis for survival: its reliability is higher than clinical signs or left ventricular ejection fraction.
Other parameters are also analyzed: anaerobic threshold, EV/VCO_2, VO_2 during recovery, VO_2 related to ventilation.

Heart valve disease

The frequency of repolarization abnormalities and of left ventricular hypertrophy explains the poor value of exercise testing in the diagnosis of an associated coronary disease. Rather the value of exercise testing lies in an objective assessment of functional tolerance in patients with valve disease claiming to be asymptomatic.

Symptomatic aortic stenosis formally contraindicates exercise testing. However, if the aortic stenosis is asymptomatic and there is discordance between ultrasound and clinical data, exercise testing can provide useful information on factors suggestive of poor prognosis: low functional capacity, abnormal blood pressure response (hypotension or low blood pressure increase during exercise), symptoms triggered by exercise, or arrhythmia.

Arrhythmia

Exercise testing is useful in exploring exercise-related symptoms and signs (syncope, palpitations, dyspnea), to specify the mechanism that triggers arrhythmia or to assess treatment efficacy.

In Wolff-Parkinson-White syndrome, permeability of the accessory pathway can be assessed. In cases of a long refractory period, the delta wave disappears during exercise, and the Wolff-Parkinson-White syndrome is benign. If the refractory period is short, pre-stimulation persists with high HR, leading to a risk of rapid atrial fibrillation and sudden death.

Exercise testing and expired gas analysis

WHAT IS VO₂?

A human being at rest, lying down and in thermal equilibrium, has an oxygen uptake of about 3.5 mL O_2/kg/min. This is the basic metabolic rate and is used as a reference. Any activity can be characterized as a multiple of this basal metabolism and can be expressed in **METs (metabolic equivalents)**.

Basal metabolism = 1 MET = 3.5 mL O_2/kg/min

VO_2 increases proportionally with exercise intensity and then plateaus - at VO_2 max - despite further increases in exercise intensity. *Maximum oxygen uptake reflects physical fitness.* These seemingly simple notions combine a number of determinants related to the muscles, heart, and respiration. On average, VO_2 max decreases by 10% per decade after the age of 20 (5% for those who exercise regularly).

PRINCIPLES, MEASURED AND CALCULATED PARAMETERS

A facial mask or mouthpiece is used to measure three parameters in the upper airways (Fig. 1 and Table I):

▶ Oxygen (O_2) content in exhaled air;

▶ Carbon dioxide (CO_2) content in exhaled air;

▶ Ventilation (VE expressed in L/min).

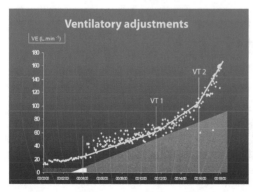

Fig. 1
Ventilatory tresholds determination of thresholds depends on the detection of two slope changes in the analysis of VO_2 kinetics.

Table I - VO$_2$: Main parameters used in clinical practice	
Parameter	**Description**
VO$_2$	VO$_2$ max is associated with specific criteria: respiratory exchange ratio > 1.1; depletion of cardiac or ventilatory reserves; blood acidosis. Norms for VO$_2$ max for sex and age.
VCO$_2$	Concentration of CO$_2$ in exhaled air increases with exercise, evidence of the combustion of energy substrates.
Ventilatory flow (VE)	Ventilatory flow rises with exercise due to an increase in respiratory rate and tidal volume.
Ventilatory equivalents	Corresponding to the number of liters of air ventilated to supply one liter of O$_2$ to the organism (Eq O$_2$ = VE/VO$_2$) and extract one liter of CO$_2$ produced (Eq CO$_2$ = VE/VCO$_2$). They are indicative of respiratory efficiency.

Respiratory quotient RQ = VCO$_2$/VO$_2$

At rest, indicates the energy pathway called into play:

RQ < 1: evidence of the preferential use of triglycerides;

RQ = 1: use of glucose;

At work, for RQ >1: there is more CO$_2$ released than O$_2$ consumed.

Exhaustion usually comes with an RQ close to 1.1.

ANAEROBIC THRESHOLD

At the onset of effort, ventilation is adapted to VO$_2$. After a certain level, a threshold is reached in ventilation and in the VE/VO$_2$ ratio, which is secondary to an increased production of CO$_2$. This anaerobic threshold is expressed by an increase in the ventilatory equivalent for oxygen (VE/VO$_2$) without any change in the ventilatory equivalent for carbon dioxide (VE/VCO$_2$).

VENTILATORY COMPENSATION POINT

At the ventilatory compensation point, respiration is no longer controlled and becomes ineffectual. This can be explained by a pH decrease (acidosis), which leads to a stimulation of VE and a threshold in VE/VCO$_2$ ratio.

LIMITS TO DETERMINING THRESHOLDS

In nearly 15% of cases, it is difficult to find significant changes in slope curves, particularly when patients are anxious before performing the test (ill-adapted ventilation).

VO$_2$ EXERCISE TEST: MAIN INDICATIONS IN CARDIOLOGY

DYSPNEA EVALUATION

Dyspnea is a frequently reported symptom which cause may be difficult to determine by history and clinical examination with the patient at rest. Pulmonary function tests are therefore done. When the diagnosis is uncertain, a VO$_2$ exercise test can reproduce functional symptoms, which can help determine the most probable cause (cardiac, pulmonary, peripheral, or central).

QUANTIFYING HEART FAILURE, AND PROGNOSIS

Aerobic capacity decrease reflects the severity and duration of heart failure. A VO$_2$ exercise test can help define treatment:

▶ When VO$_2$ max is less than 10 mL/kg/min, a heart transplant is recommended.

▶ When VO$_2$ max is between 10 and 18 mL/kg/min, treatment will depend on the ventilatory equivalent for carbon dioxide (VE/VCO$_2$), which reflects central regulation abnormalities.

If patients with heart failure are not keen to exercise, the anaerobic threshold can be used, as it correlates well with VO$_2$ max.

TREATMENT FOLLOW-UP

Improvement in cardiocirculatory and ventilatory data indicates that treatment is efficient.

MANAGING CARDIAC REHABILITATION

The aim of cardiac rehabilitation is not only to improve cardiocirculatory and ventilatory measurements, but also to increase patient autonomy. This requires raising of the anaerobic threshold. Current protocols for cardiac rehabilitation use power and heart rate corresponding to the anaerobic threshold to establish training programs.

The efficiency of rehabilitation is assessed in terms of:

Maximum power: VO₂ max; % of the norm
Gain expressed in watts and in percentage of initial data.

Anaerobic threshold: Capacities expressed in VO₂ (mL/kg/min) and in METs
Gain expressed in watts and in percentage of initial power.

Ventilation: Decrease in respiratory rate (RR) and ventilatory equivalent for O₂ (VE/VCO₂) and ventilatory equivalent for CO₂ (VE/VCO₂) for the same amount of exercise.
Taking ECG and blood pressure into account.

Improvement in HR/W and BP/W ratios.
These values, plus other test findings, help cardiologists to determine a patient's capacities and prospects of returning to work.

SPECIFIC CASES: ARRHYTHMIA AND PACEMAKER FOLLOW-UP;
POST-TRANSPLANTATION FOLLOW-UP

In such cases VO₂ exercise testing is designed not only to collect cardiovascular data, but also to determine objective functional capacities (Table II).

Table II - Main indications for determination of VO_2	
Dyspnea evaluation	VO_2 usually indicates the probable cause (cardiac, pulmonary, or central)
Evaluation of the degree of cardiac insufficiency and prognosis	Guides therapeutic indications, especially concerning transplantation
Cardiac insufficiency: treatment follow-up	Objective assessment of treatment effectiveness
Cardiac rehabilitation	Primary evaluation and objective assessment of progress
Sports medicine	Primary assessment, guide to choice of activities and their intensity
Social medicine	Objective determination of the patient's degree of autonomy and functional capacities
Preoperative evaluation	Helps to manage perioperative risk

RELEVANT PARAMETERS IN STANDARD PRACTICE

SPORTS MEDICINE

▶ **Subjects starting sports:**
- Initial VO$_2$ max, used as a reference for follow-up;
- Anaerobic threshold representing exercise intensity in endurance.

▶ **Subjects who exercise regularly:**
- VO$_2$ max showing maximum capacities and maximum aerobic speed or maximum aerobic power, depending on the ergometer used (treadmill or cycle);
- Anaerobic threshold below which no additional progress will be made with further training;
- Ventilatory compensation point indicating tolerance to endurance exercise.

▶ **Highly trained athletes:**
VO$_2$ max; anaerobic threshold; ventilatory compensation point; maximum aerobic speed; time limit (how long exercise is tolerated at VO$_2$ max).

Choose activities whose energy cost is compatible with VO$_2$ exercise test results.

SOCIAL MEDICINE

Anaerobic threshold can be used to estimate a patient's degree of autonomy, whether he or she should stay at home, and the kind of home help needed (nurse, domestic help, etc.) according to the underlying disease. Capacities below 85% of the norm for sex and age are a sign of moderately impaired capacity; below 60% indicates severe impairment.

OCCUPATIONAL MEDICINE

Anaerobic threshold, plus the results of specific cardiovascular exams, is used to measure a patient's functional capacity and to decide on a return to a suitable job. In cases of incapacity, the level of disability is based on VO$_2$ max expressed as a percentage of the norm for sex and age.

PREOPERATIVE EVALUATION

Cardiovascular (ECG, BP), ventilatory (TV, VE max, HR) and metabolic (VO$_2$ max or VO$_2$ max expressed as a percentage of the norm) functions can help predict how well the perioperative period will go. Abnormalities should be properly managed.

PULMONOLOGY

Pulmonary function tests should precede and follow VO_2 exercise testing, which should be carried out with the patient taking his or her usual treatments. Changes in respiratory rate, tidal volume, arterial oxygen saturation, and dyspnea can be used to estimate a patient's capacities and limits.

PRESCRIBING EXERCISE FOR OVERWEIGHT PATIENTS

When exercising at an intensity of less than 50% of VO_2 max, the body uses fatty acids as a source of energy, particularly when there are no simple carbohydrates.

As a result, sustained, low-intensity physical activities mobilize the body's fat reserves. VO_2 exercise test results can be used to define such activities and their intensity.

ASSESSMENT PRIOR TO HEART TRANSPLANT

VO_2 max expressed as an absolute value (*cf. above*) and as a percentage of the norm is recognized to be helpful in predicting prognosis. Anaerobic threshold is more often reached, and is of the same prognostic value. It documents the degree of autonomy and is used to determine rehabilitation. It is important to measure the fat percentage (skinfold caliper or impedance measurement). Oxygen uptake during exercise occurs in muscles, while the results are based on total mass. As a result, results are lower in subjects with a high percentage of body fat. This is an important argument that could motivate obese patients with heart failure to lose weight before making a final decision.

CONCLUSION

Exercise testing with expired gas analysis provides a comprehensive assessment of a subject and his or her limits during exercise, rather than at rest. Its use requires a thorough knowledge of physiology and a rigorous technical approach.

Radionuclide myocardial perfusion imaging

INTRODUCTION

Radionuclide myocardial perfusion imaging is a complement to exercise testing. The rationale for combining exercise testing and myocardial perfusion imaging is the so-called "ischemic cascade", which can be summarized as follows: During ischemia (Table I):

- Myocardial perfusion is altered first and is : studied using isotopic techniques;
- With a 70% decrease in myocardial perfusion, wall motion is altered: this can be studied using isotopic and ultrasound techniques;
- Repolarization abnormalities occur later: they are analyzed by exercise testing;
- Angina is the tip of the iceberg.

Isotopic techniques produce images of myocardial perfusion, both at rest and after an ischemic stimulation (such as effort). Briefly, one talks about ischemia when perfusion is abnormal during exercise but not at rest. Necrosis, or infarction, is characterized by abnormal perfusion both during exercise and at rest.

Table I - The ischemic cascade	
Hierarchy of abnormalities	**Evaluation**
Alteration of myocardial perfusion	Radionuclide imaging
Regional kinetics anomaly	Ultrasonography
Electrical anomalies	ECG
Angina	Clinical

Remarks

Myocardial perfusion imaging using single-photon emission computed tomography (SPECT) has existed since the 1970s, and in the 1980s experienced a rapid expansion with the development of tomographic techniques. Subsequently, the technique was synchronized with electrocardiography, thereby enabling quantitative analysis of ventricular function.

About 10 million myocardial SPECTs were performed in the United States in 2008. Hybrid techniques, combining a single-photon (SPECT) or double-photon (PET) camera and a CT scanning device, are paving the way to provide anatomic and functional information. New cardiac imaging techniques are physiological (in tandem with exercise testing), quick and comprehensive: they provide objective and rational data for therapeutic decision-making.

SINGLE-PHOTON EMISSION COMPUTED TOMOGRAPHY

▶ **A tracer** is a substance with a strong affinity for myocardial cells receiving a normal blood supply. A tracer emits photons (atoms emit only one photon, hence the term "single-photon").

▶ **A gamma camera** analyzes the photons emitted by the tracer.

▶ **Emission imaging** means that the radiation emitted by the organ is detected by a camera outside the body. (Radiology is imaging by transmission: the X-ray tube emits radiation that goes through the patient, then interacts with the detector.) Hence the term single-photon emission computed tomography or SPECT. Some tracers emit two photons; they are called positrons and are recorded with positron emission tomography (PET) (Fig. 1).

Remarks

Gamma radiation emission is isotropic, ie, photons are emitted in all directions. Since the head detector is flat, only a small proportion of gamma rays reaches it. For photons to interact effectively with the detector, they must not only be emitted in the direction of the gamma camera head, but must also reach it (without being absorbed by the thorax or the myocardium and without being deviated) and arrive strictly perpendicular to the surface of the camera (current collimators stop other photons).

This is why, in practice, only 1/10 000 emitted photons on average effectively serves to create an image. Recent advances should considerably improve the efficiency of detectors by changing their morphology, nature, and collimation. A 10-fold improvement is expected, which should quarter acquisition times and double image resolution.

WHAT ISCHEMIC STIMULUS SHOULD BE CHOSEN PRIOR TO MYOCARDIAL SPECT?

This is an essential step in myocardial perfusion imaging: the greater the stimulation, the higher the test's sensitivity (Table II).

EXERCISE TESTING IS THE BEST WAY TO INDUCE ISCHEMIA:

- It is physiological;
- It provides invaluable information about physical fitness (with high prognostic value), blood pressure, arrhythmia, and, of course, ECG modifications;
- It can be performed on a cycle ergometer or treadmill.

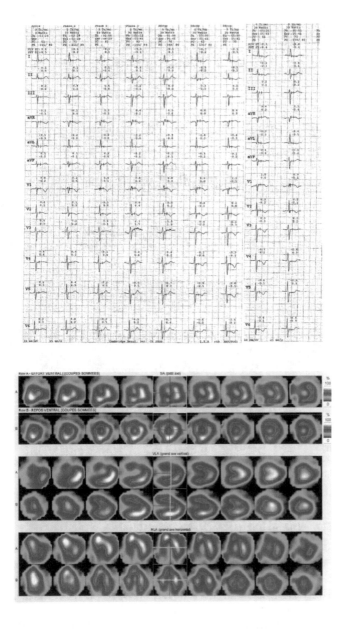

Fig. 1 - Lateral ST depression with intraventricular conduction disturbance in a patient with scintigraphic evidence of antero-septal ischemia.

Table II - Provocation tests for ischemia		
	Advantages	**Disadvantages**
Exercise test	Physiological	Loss of sensitivity if submaximal
Dipyridamole	Possible in subjects unable to exercise; reference test in case of LBBB, pacemaker	Less sensitive than a maximum exercise test; frequent adverse drug reactions
Dipyridamole + effort	Physiological. Equal to a maximum exercise test.	?

Remarks

When the exercise test is submaximal, it is possible to overlook myocardial ischemia, even when combined with radionuclide imaging.

DIPYRIDAMOLE ALONE

Mechanism of action: (Distal) arteriolar vasodilation generates a 500% increase in coronary blood flow in a normal subject. When there is significant stenosis, blood flow increase is blunted downstream the stenosis, but remains normal in disease-free regions. Isotopic techniques use this difference.

Dipyridamole also has a vasodilating action on the systemic arterial system resulting in a blood pressure decrease that depends on the individual. This decrease in BP generates a moderate heart rate acceleration.

Protocol: 0.56 mg.kg^{-1} in 4 minutes, possibly with an additional half dose. The response varies from one individual to another.

Indications : Use in situations where exercise is impossible and when there is a spontaneous (LBBB) or induced intraventricular disorder (pacemaker). Asynchronous contraction of the interventricular septum can lead to relative hypoperfusion of the septum in cases of short diastole, ie, when the heart rate is high, during exercise, for example. For this reason, it is generally preferable to use a dipyridamole-only stimulation in these cases.

Contraindications: Asthmatic subjects or patients with severe chronic obstructive lung disease, hypotensive subjects or those with a significant carotid stenosis. Careful use is recommended in cases of aortic stenosis, congestive heart failure, and pulmonary arterial hypertension.

Adverse drug reactions: Headache, hypotension, vertigo, nausea, pain not corresponding to angina. Death 0.95/10 000, nonfatal myocardial infarction 1.8/10 000, severe bronchospasm 1.2/10 000, transient ischemic attack 1.2/10 000.

Antidote: Aminophylline.

THE COMBINATION DYPYRIDAMOLE + STRESS TESTING IS WIDELY USED since it produces an ischemic stimulation equivalent to that of a maximum stress test.

OTHER WAYS TO INDUCE CARDIOVASCULAR STRESS
These are rarely used:
- In some asthmatic subjects, dobutamine can be used (severe side effects - ventricular tachycardia, flush, headaches, tremor, dyspnea, etc. - reported in up to 80% of patients in some series);
- Atropine and Isuprel® are very rarely used.

TRACERS USED FOR MYOCARDIAL SPECT

Whatever the type of perfusion tracer used, it is injected at peak exercise or at the moment of maximum vasodilation when pharmacologic agents are used (7 minutes after the onset of perfusion for dipyridamole, 6 minutes for adenosine) (Table III and Fig. 2).

Table III - Comparative characteristics of tracers used for myocardial SPECT		
	Advantages	**Disadvantages**
Thallium-201	The most physiological: high myocardial uptake, low subdiaphragmatic uptake	Low-energy photons: image quality sometimes suboptimal
MIBI and other technetium-labeled tracers	High-energy photons: image quality usually better than with thallium. More precise ejection fraction assessment.	Lower myocardial uptake than thallium. Subdiaphragmatic uptake can be troublesome. Production of 99mTc cyclotron-dependent.

Remarks

Ideally, myocardial uptake of a perfusion tracer should be proportional to coronary blood flow. This has proven to be true only for labeled albumin microspheres that cannot be intravenously injected (they are stopped by pulmonary capillaries). Clinically used tracers show a plateau effect: for values exceeding twice the initial blood flow (recorded during exercise and after pharmacologic stimulation), myocardial tracer uptake increases less than coronary flow.

This reduces sensitivity for detecting coronary stenoses and limits quantification of absolute blood flow.

THALLIUM-201

Historically, thallium-201 was the first tracer to be used routinely. It plateaus less than technetium-labeled tracers, which makes it more sen-

THE SEQUENCE OF EVENTS DURING RADIONUCLIDE IMAGING

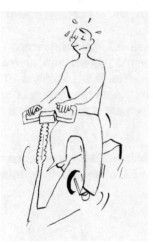

Stress testing

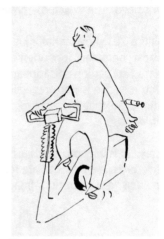

Tracer injection

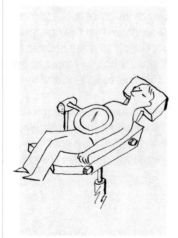

Image acquisition

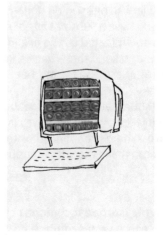

Image processing

Fig. 2 - Series of figures showing the sequence of events during radionuclide imaging.

sitive for detecting coronary stenoses. However, the energy of emitted photons (79 keV) causes more attenuation than technetium-labeled tracers, whose photons give off more energy (140 keV).

Thallium-201 has a long half-life - (half-life = time after which half the atoms have disintegrated) - preventing the use of large doses.

Thallium-201 shows what is known as a redistribution phenomenon: the contrast between low-uptake ischemic regions and normal-uptake disease-free regions disappears after a few hours. Thallium-201 uptake during exercise is not irreversible: exchanges between cells and blood continue, so that the ischemic phenomenon progressively disappears after exercise.

This explains why protocols using thallium-201 as tracer necessarily start with exercise testing and are followed 3 hours later by imaging at rest (known as "redistribution" images).

Technetium-labeled tracers

These tracers do not have a redistribution effect. An initial exercise protocol can be used, followed by imaging at rest, or imaging at rest can be followed by imaging during exercise. In either case, the second image should have a substantially higher tracer dose than the first, so as not to be contaminated by the first injection. Owing to large hepatic and vesicular uptake of these tracers, images should not be recorded immediately after exercise testing, but rather 15 minutes to 1 hour afterwards.

The short half-life of technetium-99m (6 hours) means larger doses can be injected, which improves image quality. Technetium-labeled tracers have a more pronounced plateau phenomenon than thallium-201, and this can make them less sensitive in detecting coronary stenoses.

Double isotope techniques

These techniques combine imaging at rest after an injection of thallium-201, followed by stress imaging after an injection of a technetium-labeled tracer. The main advantage of this expensive method, which is mainly used in the US, is that it significantly reduces the total time of the protocol.

WHAT PATIENTS SHOULD KNOW WHEN MAKING AN APPOINTMENT FOR MYOCARDIAL SPECT

SHOULD I HAVE AN EMPTY STOMACH?
No. Performing an exercise test on an empty stomach could cause a vasovagal episode and hypoglycemia. Have a normal breakfast, but replace coffee or tea (which contain xanthic bases, antidotes to dipyridamole) with fruit juice.

SHOULD I INTERUPT ANGINA TREATMENT?
It depends:
If the test is being done to diagnose ischemic cardiopathy, it is advantageous to interrupt treatment, especially if it consists of beta-blockers (although the combination of dipyridamole + exercise is not very sensitive to the "maximal" character of the exercise test).

If the test is being done to assess a known and treated ischemic cardiopathy, treatment should not be interrupted.

HOW IS THE EXAMINATION DONE?
Centers using thallium-201 start by exercise testing, followed by the first round of imaging. This first step lasts 35 to 45 minutes. The images at rest are recorded about 3 hours later. This second step lasts 15 to 20 minutes.
Centers using a technetium-labeled tracer start with imaging at rest, about 30 minutes after the injection. This first step lasts about 50 minutes, after which an exercise test is performed, followed by imaging after a wait of 30 to 60 minutes. The second step lasts for about 90 minutes. It is also possible to start with imaging during exercise, which, if normal, eliminates the need for the second step.

TYPICAL MYOCARDIAL SPECT REPORT

REASONS FOR THE TEST
- Initial diagnosis of coronary disease: describe symptoms;
- Follow-up of a known coronary artery disease: key moments (infarction, revascularization);
- Describe risk factors;
- Specify the context: taking up sport again, peripheral arteriopathy, at-risk profession, etc.

ISCHEMIA-PROVOCATION TEST
Protocol
- Exercise test: method (treadmill or cycle ergometer), protocol;
- Pharmacologic stimulation: product, dose.

Results
Reasons for stopping the test, exercise level reached, percentage of MPHR, symptoms during the test, ECG changes, rhythm disorders, BP profile.

MYOCARDIAL SPECT
Protocol
- Tracer: product, injected activity;
- Imaging: patient's position in relation to the detector (prone or supine), duration, conditions for rest imaging (or "redistribution" if thallium).

Results
- Myocardial perfusion: uptake defects after stimulation and at rest (location, depth, size, reversibility);
- Gated SPECT ventricular function: global ejection fraction, regional kinetics, assessment of right ventricular function.

GENERAL CONCLUSION
Should provide a comprehensive review of exercise test and SPECT data:
- Level of effort reached;
- Ischemia (location, extent) with or without clinical and/or electrocardiographic abnormalities;
- Infarction (location, size);
- Left ventricular function, myocardial viability.

Signatures of the doctor(s).

CLINICAL VALUE OF MYOCARDIAL SPECT

COMPARISON WITH CORONARY ANGIOGRAPHY

The diagnostic performances of myocardial SPECT have historically been expressed in terms of sensitivity, specificity, negative and positive predictive value, and diagnostic precision with regard to coronary angiography, the gold standard for coronary stenosis (Table IV). SPECT performances vary significantly depending on studies, primarily due to methodological differences: study population (prevalence of diabetes and obesity, for example), tracers used, radionuclide imaging equipment, visual or automated interpretation of images, coronary angiography criteria (50% or 70% reduction in luminal diameter), etc.

On average, the combination of ECG and SPECT data usually provide results in the range of 90% for sensitivity and 85% for specificity, but these results depend greatly on the size and expertise of the center performing the isotopic examination.

Table IV - Diagnostic value of myocardial SPECT (with reference to coronary angiography)
Sensitivity: 85% to 94%
Specificity: 70% to 90%
Diagnostic precision: 70% to 96%

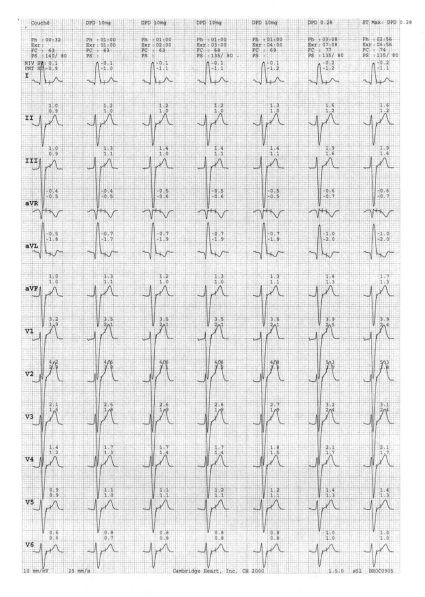

Fig. 3 - Apical ischemia with no ECG abnormality during exercise test.

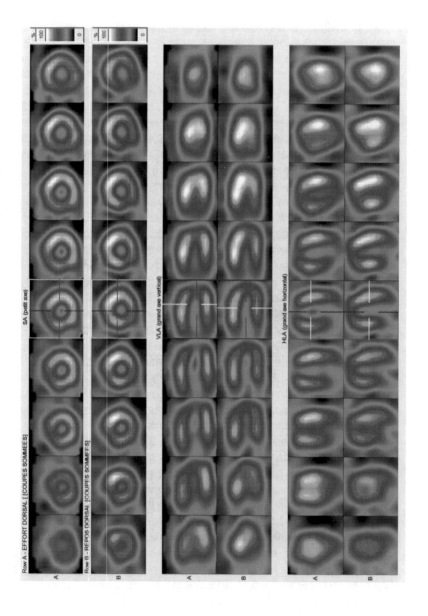

Why myocardial SPECT and coronary angiography are not a perfect match.

The nature of the comparison

Myocardial SPECT is a functional examination most often performed during exercise, allowing for a semi-quantitative assessment of myocardial perfusion, while coronary angiography is an anatomic examination that visualizes the lumen of large coronary vessels at rest. The correlation between the degree of stenosis, visually assessed on an angiogram, and its functional impact, determined by SPECT, has been the subject of numerous studies. It remains imperfect for several reasons:

- The exact quantification of the degree of stenosis ("tight" or not) remains difficult: coronary angiography is a "projection" technique juxtaposing various elements that are crossed by the X-ray beam. In a 3-mm diameter vessel, the difference between a 40% stenosis and a 60% stenosis is 0.6 mm, which is a very thin gap, even for a trained eye;

- Expressing severity of stenosis using the percentage diameter has the advantage of simplicity, but also serious disadvantages: it looks neither at the length of the narrowing nor at the diameter of the native vessel. A 50% stenosis leaves a residual lumen of 2-mm in a 4-mm diameter vessel and of 0.75-mm in a 1.5-mm vessel: the hemodynamic impact is clearly different, but the two stenoses are assessed as 50%;

- Most stenoses are off-center, asymmetrical, and have a disease-free lining. As a general rule, this segment retains significant vasomotricity, especially during exercise, where some stenoses worsen and others dilate. Coronary endothelium plays a dominant role in this "dynamic" nature of stenoses. It also has a major prognostic impact: subjects whose endothelial function is normal have a more favorable prognosis than those whose endothelial function is altered. This probably explains why functional data are usually more informative about prognosis than anatomical data: during exercise, endothelial function influences the results, which are therefore a combination of anatomical and biological data. A 50% stenosis with a normal endothelium will dilate during exercise, resulting in a 40% stenosis and no ischemia. Since endothelial function is normal, the risk of plaque rupture and acute coronary syndrome is low. Conversely, if endothelial function is abnormal, the stenosis will worsen during exercise and become a 60% stenosis resulting in myocardial ischemia. This abnormal endothelial function exposes the patient to plaque rupture and carries a higher risk. Both stenoses are anatomically identical at 50% in this example, but their biological nature is different and can be revealed during stress, so that one produces ischemia and is a high-risk stenosis, while the other is not.

SPECT artifacts

Artifacts are the second explanation for the differences noted between coronary angiography and myocardial SPECT. It is essential to distinguish between false positives and false negatives.

The term false positive is used to describe a defect that mimics a perfusion abnormality. False positives reduce the technique's specificity. The development of advanced detectors and the nuclear physician's degree of expertise have a significant impact on the number of artifacts, which are usually explained by the patient's body absorbing an excessive number of photons, especially in overweight patients. This type of artifact can be limited by:

- A maximum intensity ischemia-induction test;
- Injection of an appropriate tracer dose;
- Sufficient acquisition time, requiring the patient to remain immobile;
- If need be, imaging in the prone position.

False negatives concern patients with a normal SPECT and a coronary angiography indicating the presence of one or several significant stenoses. These patients have a normal coronary reserve and follow-up indicates that their prognosis is similar to that of patients with no stenosis. This most often concerns patients who have developed a coronary collateral network or still have good endothelial function. The rare patients who have diffuse ischemia are generally identified by positive clinical and/or electrical characteristics on the exercise test, a decrease in ejection fraction and/or an increase in pulmonary uptake of the tracer during exercise.

Prognosis

Combining exercise testing with myocardial SPECT is the noninvasive technique that gives the best prognostic information in ischemic heart disease: the greater the perfusion abnormalities, the higher the risk.

These results have been documented in several thousand patients and demonstrate that, by combining exercise testing with SPECT, it is possible to differentiate between low-risk subjects, for whom optimal treatment combines dietary preventive measures, physical activity, and drug treatment, and higher-risk subjects, who should benefit from revascularization.

Risk assessment of SPECT is precise enough for therapeutic decision-making, especially between medical treatment alone or combined with revascularization.

WHAT IS THE VALUE OF A NORMAL MYOCARDIAL SPECT?

A normal myocardial SPECT is linked to a very low risk of cardiac events, below 1% annually. This result has been confirmed by numerous studies, covering about 40 000 patients. The risk for a patient with a normal SPECT and "significant" stenoses (50%–70%) is between 1% and 2% per year.

A normal SPECT is valuable because, compared with other techniques, it analyzes the myocardial perfusion, the first abnormal parameter during ischemia. Self-regulating mechanisms protect the contraction of the myocardium, so that regional kinetics - on the other hand - remain normal for a long time: a 70% reduction of myocardial perfusion is needed to observe regional function abnormalities.

Other advantages of isotopes are that SPECT techniques are not very patient-dependent, and can usually be performed after a maximum stress test (the combination of dipyridamole plus effort). A submaximal test leads to a decrease in the sensitivity of any imaging technique, and consequently reduces its value.

Statistically, a normal SPECT remains valid for two years. In patients with diabetes or atrial fibrillation, this duration should be shortened.

THE RELATIVE ROLE OF MYOCARDIAL SPECT AND MULTIDETECTOR COMPUTED TOMOGRAPHY

Multidetector computed tomography (MDCT) has an excellent negative predictive value when the test is of good quality (slow and regular heart rate, absence of stent or calcifications). As a result, MDCT, which irradiation dose rate is high, is indicated for patients with a low probability of coronary disease, but for whom one needs a formal diagnosis.

In patients with stenoses that look tight on MDCT, it is recommended to check their functional importance before resorting to coronary angiography.

The spatial resolution of MDCT is about 0.45 mm (*versus* 0.2 mm for coronary angiography), which means an error of ± 20% in a 3 mm coronary artery. Stenosis assessed as 50% by MDCT may therefore correspond to stenosis between 30% and 70% on coronary angiography. MDCT does not currently have a high enough resolution to assess the exact degree of a coronary stenosis. This test is not recommended in the follow-up of stents.

Fewer than half of subjects with stenoses that look tight on MDCT are ischemic by myocardial SPECT. This is important in treatment choice (medical treatment alone or combined with revascularization), since only patients who are really ischemic benefit from revascularization.

COST EFFECTIVENESS

The cost effectiveness of myocardial SPECT has been documented for years in the United States, where it has been shown that its rational use, mainly in populations with an intermediate risk, noticeably reduces costs. More recently, cost effectiveness studies have shown that despite higher up-front costs, SPECT is more cost effective than stress echocardiography.

This is because normal stress echocardiography is less accident-free than radionuclide imaging (<1% annual accidents after normal SPECT, *versus* 4% to 8% after normal stress echocardiography) and because 20% to 30% of stress echos are of "suboptimal" quality, even in the most skilled hands. When reassessing the resulting costs, radionuclide imaging remains unsurpassed in terms of cost effectiveness due to the great reliability of its results, as assessed in tens of thousands of patients.

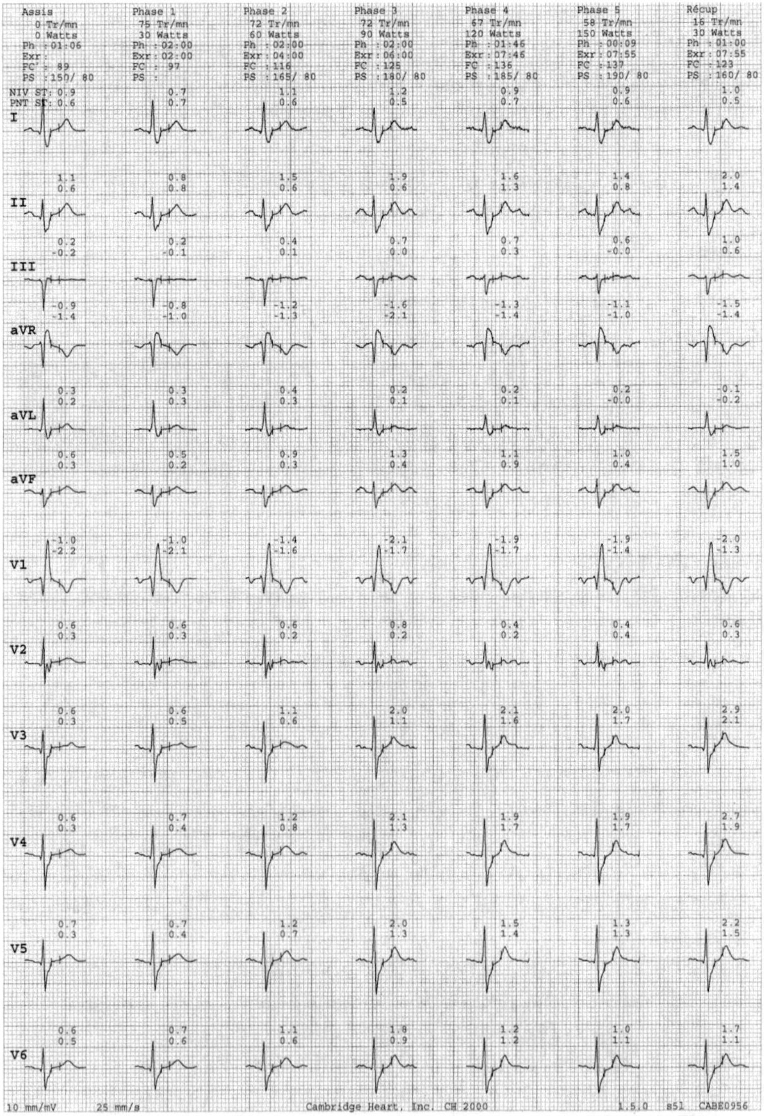

Fig. 4 - Large infero-apical ischemia with normal ECG during exercise test.

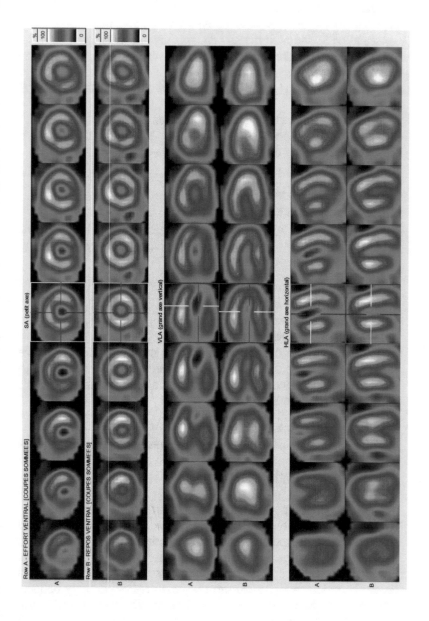

MAJOR INDICATIONS FOR MYOCARDIAL SPECT

BORDERLINE EXERCISE TEST

In 15% to 20% of cases, exercise test results are borderline:

- Ascending ST-segment depression less than one millimeter;
- Atypical repolarization modifications concerning the T wave or recorded only during recovery;
- Submaximal test (in terms of MPHR or with regard to the target physical capacity);
- Test clinically positive but with no repolarization modification;
- Test difficult or impossible to read: LBBB, right bundle branch block, infarction sequelae, repolarization disorders on the initial ECG, etc.

A borderline exercise test is one of the best indications for myocardial SPECT.

EXERCISE TESTING NOT POSSIBLE

Some patients with orthopedic or neurological diseases, for example, cannot perform the exercise test, and only pharmacologic stress testing is possible.

INTERMEDIATE PREVALENCE

When the probability of coronary disease is:

- neither low (young subject, asymptomatic or few symptoms);
- nor high (65-year-old patient with typical angina).

Exercise testing is of limited value (3 false-positive or false-negative results out of 10 examinations). Combining exercise testing with myocardial SPECT can be recommended as a first-line strategy in this intermediate risk population.

ASSESSMENT OF LESIONS SEEN ON MDCT

MDCT does not provide a functional assessment of atheromatous lesions, even when the stenosis looks tight. Myocardial SPECT combined with exercise testing plays an important role in this situation.

THE ROLE OF MYOCARDIAL SPECT IN THERAPEUTIC DECISION-MAKING

Numerous studies published between 1998 and 2007 have demonstrated that - on average - percutaneous revascularization is not superior to medical treatment in stable coronary disease. When SPECT results are included in the decision-making process, it is noted that percutaneous revascularization tends to worsen the prognosis of coronary patients who are not ischemic. This is because patients with normal SPECT have an annual risk below 1%, whereas percutaneous revascularization itself carries a risk of about 1%, to which subsequent risks must be added (sudden stent occlusion, restenosis, and accidents linked to the use of anticoagulant and antiplatelet agents or to their interruption). On the other hand, if there is significant myocardial ischemia (more than 10% of the myocardium), the risk is higher than 2%, and revascularization significantly and objectively improves the prognosis.

Angioplasty improves prognosis in cases of significant ischemia. Patients with coronary stenosis but without significant ischemia - and they are numerous - benefit from treatments that combine dietary measures, physical activity, and a drug regimen.

Significant coronary stenosis

• *Ischemia of more than 10% of the myocardium: angioplasty (stenting) improves prognosis;*

• *Absence of ischemia or minimal ischemia (collateral circulation, preserved endothelial function, stenosis that is, in fact, not very tight): stenting does not provide any improvement over medical treatment and can even be harmful in stable coronary disease.*

FOLLOW-UP AFTER INFARCTION AND AFTER REVASCULARIZATION

Stenting carries a risk of restenosis (between 10% to 20% in the first year). Exercise testing alone and MDCT show poor results for the diagnosis of restenosis. Myocardial SPECT currently remains the best noninvasive test for diagnosis of restenosis or more precisely for the diagnosis of recurrence of ischemia, in the revascularized region or in another region. All available studies show that revascularized patients with a normal myocardial SPECT have a risk that is near zero.

After infarction:

• If the patient has been revascularized, the short-term issue is the detection of restenosis (see above). In the longer term, progression of lesions in the whole coronary arterial tree defines prognosis. The advantage of myocardial SPECT is that the infarction scar does not impede the detection of recurrent ischemia. Combining exercise testing with SPECT also provides information about physical fitness and ejection fraction during exercise, which are essential data for treatment follow-up. The demonstration of residual ischemia by radionuclide imaging indicates an increased risk of progression and is a good indication for coronary angiography;

- If the patient has not been revascularized, SPECT can highlight possible perinecrotic or distant residual ischemia;
- If left ventricular function is altered and revascularization is being considered, myocardial viability should be evaluated.

LBBB, PACEMAKER

Spontaneous or artificial (pacemaker) conduction disorders create an asynchronism in ventricular contraction. The interventricular septum shifts phases in relation to other regions of the ventricle.

During exercise, heart rate increases, diastole duration decreases and septal kinetics may show phase opposition with other regions of the ventricle. Septal perfusion can therefore be compromised by a "crushing" of the septum that results from the asynchronous contraction. In these conditions, it is better to opt for an induction test that does not modify heart rate (dipyridamole, rather than exercise).

PERIPHERAL ARTERIOPATHY

Clinical data and the type of intervention are normally enough to determine the risk and the approach to be adopted. Myocardial SPECT is best indicated in subjects at intermediate risk (eg, 60-year-old patient who requires surgery for abdominal aorta aneurysm and presents numerous risk factors). International recommendations advocate the management of coronary problems separately from surgery. Significant ischemia (more than 10% of the myocardium) is an indication for coronary angiography/revascularization. The absence of ischemia or an ischemia that is not very convincing is an indication for drug management and should not postpone surgery.

ASTHMA

Clinical asthma is a contraindication to dipyridamole, and exercise alone should be used. Dobutamine can be used if the exercise test is too submaximal. With radionuclide imaging, right ventricular dysfunction - frequent in chronic lung disease - may give a particular appearance to the septum, which should not be confused with ischemia. Increased pulmonary uptake is frequent. Here too, this does not necessarily correspond to left ventricular dysfunction (Table V).

Table V - Major indications for myocardial SPECT	
Indications	**Remarks**
Borderline exercise test	SPECT is most often decisive
Exercise test impossible	Dipyridamole test is used as a substitute for exercise
LBBB, pacemaker, Wolff-Parkinson-White syndrome	Dipyridamole test prevents septum false positives
Intermediate coronary disease prevalence	The clinical value of the exercise test associated with radionuclide imaging is superior to that of the exercise test alone
After stenting	Combining exercise testing with radionuclide imaging is more sensitive and specific than exercise testing alone
After infarction	ST-segment depression during exercise has no formal value: radionuclide imaging indicates residual ischemia
Peripheral arteriopathy	Exercise testing is often submaximal: dipyridamole + exercise testing is recommended
Asthma	Dipyridamole is contraindicated
Assessment of documented lesions on multidetector computed tomography	Less than half the lesions considered to be "significant" on multidetector computed tomography result in ischemia

VENTRICULAR DYSFUNCTION, CONGESTIVE HEART FAILURE, MYOCARDIAL HYPERTROPHY

Myocardial impairment that reaches the stage of clinical heart failure or ventricular dysfunction may be associated with impairment of the distal coronary circulation, resulting in an ischemic appearance even in the absence of proximal coronary lesions.

In the case of left ventricular dysfunction, radionuclide imaging is a sensitive but not very specific exam that is of great value if its findings are normal. If radionuclide imaging indicates an ischemic appearance, this might indicate an impaired distal coronary circulation or an authentic proximal coronary lesion. This frequently justifies diagnostic coronary angiography.

Myocardial hypertrophy does not really change radionuclide imaging sensitivity or specificity. The only slight difference to consider is that gated SPECT techniques may underestimate the ejection fraction.
When there is diffuse subendocardial hypoperfusion—this occurs in some forms of myocardial hypertrophy—perfusion images may show an artificially enlarged ventricular cavity, which can distort the ejection fraction calculation based on the contouring of the perfusion images.

MYOCARDIAL VIABILITY

Historically, PET with 18FDG has been the gold standard for assessing myocardial viability. While the metabolism of normal myocardial cells is based on fatty acids, hypoperfused but living cells use glucose, and a viable myocardium has a significant glucose uptake at rest.

As PET equipment is rare, alternative techniques have been developed. "Rest thallium" (or rest sestamibi), after administration of nitrates, provides a satisfactory answer in terms of viability, and is more sensitive than echocardiography, but less specific.
The difference resides in the fact that radionuclide imaging assesses the presence of residual metabolism, while echocardiography indicates contractile reserve. The results recently obtained by late-enhancement MRI make this new technique a credible alternative to PET (Table VI).

Table VI - Myocardial viability: available techniques		
	Advantages	**Disadvantages**
PET	Precision	Availability, cost
Rest thallium	Sensitivity	Specificity
Ultrasound	Specificity	Sensitivity, operator-dependent
MRI	Sensitivity	Nonspecific late enhancement

WHAT SHOULD BE DONE WITH MYOCARDIAL SPECT RESULTS?

In practice, three situations are possible (Table VII):

▶ Normal myocardial SPECT findings

A normal result is of high value and can be enough to put an end to testing. The risk of cardiac events is less than 1% per year. In the future, additional information about preclinical coronary atherosclerosis might be recommended (calcium scoring) to refine risk factor management.

Table VII - What should be done with radionuclide myocardial perfusion imaging results?		
Normal SPECT	**Positive SPECT (more than 10% of ischemic myocardium)**	**Intermediate situation**
Clinical follow-up	Coronary angiography	Low risk: clinical follow-up (calcium scoring?)
Discussion: calcium scoring?		High risk: diagnostic coronary angiography?

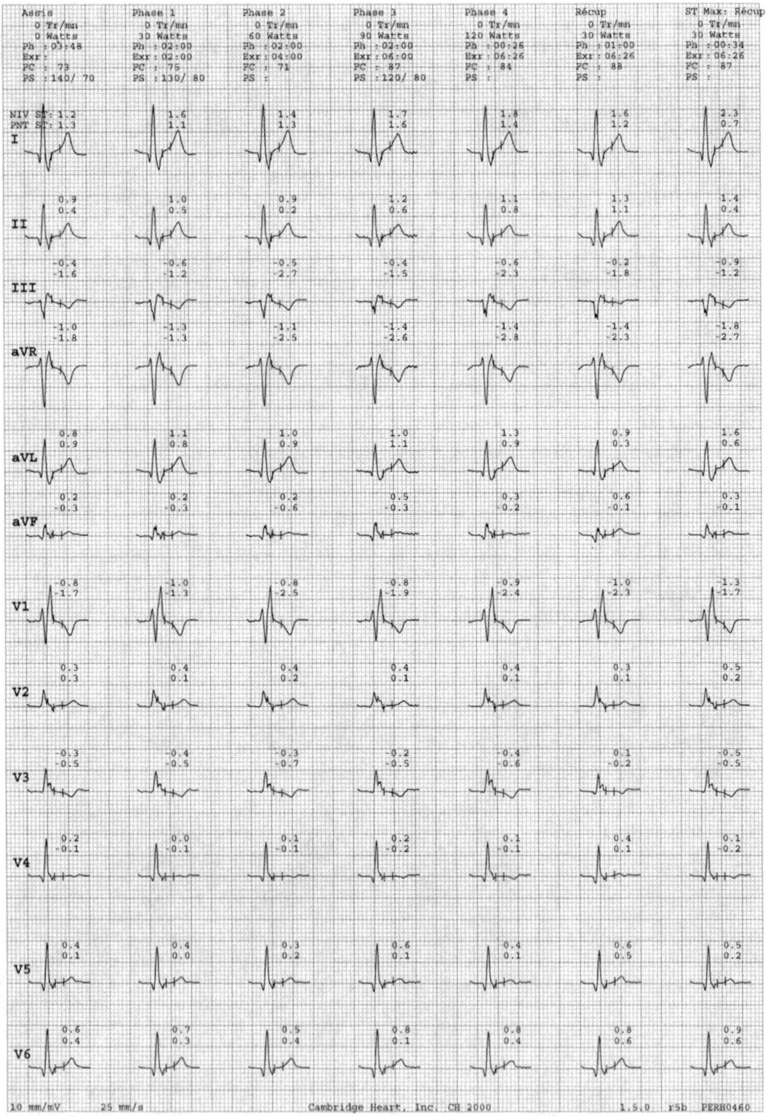

Fig. 5 - Large inferior ischemia with no ECG alteration at stress.

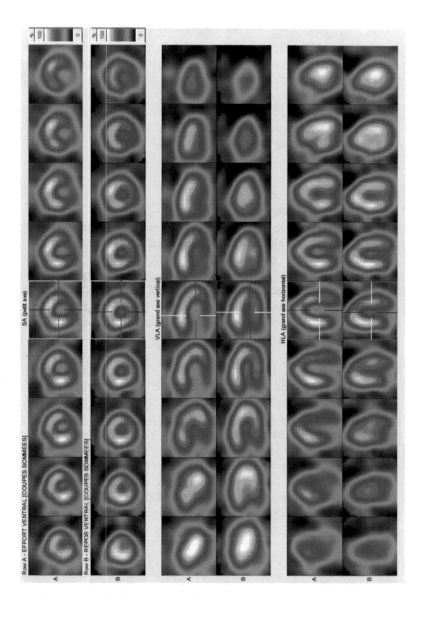

▶ **Unquestionable "significant" myocardial ischemia**
(affecting more than 10% of the myocardium). The risk is high (more than 2% per year) and justifies coronary angiography.

▶ **Intermediate situation**
Age, risk factors, exercise capacity, ventricular function, and functional signs should be considered. A simple follow-up may be enough if the risk is low (for example, a woman under the age of 60 with atypical chest pain and preserved physical capacity). If the risk seems high (man aged 70 with diabetes and reduced physical capacity), diagnostic coronary angiography may be indicated.

THE FUTURE

POSITRON EMISSION TOMOGRAPHY (PET)

As the use of PET spreads (it is a key tool used routinely in oncology), it may in the future be possible to use it in ordinary clinical cardiology. The half-life of most positron-emitting elements (^{11}C, ^{15}O, ^{13}N) is extremely short and a cyclotron is needed, so such elements cannot be used outside of research centers. The physical characteristics of other elements (^{18}F, ^{82}Rb), however enable their use in any PET center.

- ^{18}FDG is the reference for the study of myocardial viability, but it also has the interesting and distinctive feature of an increased uptake in ischemia;
- ^{18}F BMS–747158-02, currently being assessed, could become the PET reference tracer, eliminating artifacts that generate false-positive results and opening the way to quantification of coronary blood flow and reserve;
- ^{82}Rb, which has had a lot of media coverage since it was introduced in the United States, is a tracer that - in fact - might not be ideal for myocardial perfusion. Its main value is that it gives usable images in patients with morbid obesity (the images obtained with thallium-201 and technetium-labeled tracers are often of poor quality in these cases). The future will tell if the clinical performance of this tracer justifies its cost.

NEW CAMERAS

The Anger camera gives remarkable clinical results, but its photon detection and spatial resolution are poor, despite long acquisition times. Two important advances are expected in 2009 and 2010:

- Semiconductor detectors known as CZT are much more efficient than current Nal crystals;
- Improved collimation and computer signal treatment improve photon detection and management and reduce diffusion "noise".

These changes will drastically reduce acquisition time (to less than 5 minutes) and improve image resolution. They will also reduce tracer doses and enable simultaneous imaging with two different tracers.

Hybrid machines

These systems combine a computed tomography scanner and a photon detector, either gamma camera (SPECT) or PET. The PET/scanner is already commonly used in oncology. In cardiology, simultaneous recording of both anatomic and functional information will help reduce costs and improve patient care. ■

Conclusion

A century after its inception, exercise testing is more present than ever. This simple diagnostic test, which reproduces a basic human function under medical control, has found innumerable diagnostic and therapeutic applications.

Exercise testing appeared 50 years before the development of coronary arteriography, and has overcome challenges and criticisms to become the gold standard in "ischemic heart disease" underscoring that myocardial ischemia is what we seek to cure.

The subsequent spread of coronary angiography has further emphasized the need for functional evaluation of the effects of stenoses, as anatomic (radiological) visualization only contains a fraction of the information: "Anatomy is not destiny"…

Today we can assess ventricular function, myocardial perfusion, and expired gas during exercise using sophisticated and sometimes complex techniques that tomorrow will be routine and basic. These techniques will guide 30-year-old women who worry about excess weight, as well as 70-year-old men dreaming of taking up sports again. ■

Achevé d'imprimer par
l'Imprimerie Vasti-Dumas - 42010 Saint-Etienne
Dépôt légal : juillet 2009
N° d'imprimeur : V002265/00

Printed in the United States
by Baker & Taylor Publisher Services

—